Ethics in Speech
and Language Therapy

Ethics in Speech and Language Therapy

Richard Body

Senior Lecturer, Department of Human Communication Sciences
University of Sheffield, UK

Lindy McAllister

Deputy Head (Teaching and Learning)
University of Queensland Medical School

and

Adjunct Associate Professor of Speech Pathology
Charles Sturt University
Australia

(W)WILEY-BLACKWELL

A John Wiley & Sons, Ltd., Publication

This edition first published 2009,
© 2009 John Wiley & Sons

Wiley-Blackwell is an imprint of John Wiley & Sons, formed by the merger of Wiley's global Scientific, Technical and Medical business with Blackwell Publishing.

Registered office: John Wiley & Sons Ltd, The Atrium, Southern Gate, Chichester,
West Sussex, PO19 8SQ, United Kingdom

Editorial office: John Wiley & Sons Ltd,
The Atrium, Southern Gate, Chichester, West Sussex, PO19 8SQ, United Kingdom

For details of our global editorial offices, for customer services and for information about how to apply for permission to reuse the copyright material in this book please see our website at www.wiley.com/wiley-blackwell.

Library of Congress Cataloging-in-Publication Data:

Ethics in speech and language therapy / edited by Richard Body, Lindy McAllister.
 p. ; cm.
Includes bibliographical references and index.
ISBN 978-0-470-05888-6 (pbk.)
1. Speech therapists – Professional ethics. 2. Speech therapy – Moral and ethical aspects. I. Body, Richard, 1955- II. McAllister, Lindy.
[DNLM: 1. Language Therapy – ethics. 2. Speech Therapy – ethics. 3. Language Disorders – therapy. 4. Speech Disorders – therapy. WL 340.2 E837 2009]
RC428.5.E843 2009
616.85′5 – dc22

2008056027

A catalogue record for this book is available from the British Library.

Typeset in 10/12 Palatino-Roman by Laserwords Private Limited, Chennai, India

1   2009

Contents

Contributors

Kartini Ahmad
Associate Professor
Head of Department of Audiology and
  Speech Sciences
Faculty of Allied Health Sciences
Universiti Kebangsaan Malaysia

Madeline Cruice
Senior Lecturer
Department of Language and
  Communication Science
City University London
UK

Judy Duchan
Professor Emeritus
State University of New York at
  Buffalo
USA

Loraine Fordham
Speech and Language Pathologist &
  Doctoral Student
Institute of Early Childhood
Macquarie University
Australia

Linda Hand
Senior Lecturer
Speech Sciences Programme
Department of Psychology
The University of Auckland
New Zealand

Celia Harding
Lecturer
Department of Language and
  Communication Science
City University London
UK

Maggie-Lee Huckabee
Senior Lecturer
Department of Communication
  Disorders
The University of Canterbury & Van
  der Veer Institute for Parkinson's and
  Brain Research
New Zealand

Julie Marshall
Senior Research Fellow
Research Institute for Health and
  Social Change &
  Senior Lecturer in Speech and
  Language Therapy
Professional Registration Department
Manchester Metropolitan University
UK

Rosemary Martino
Assistant Professor
Graduate Department of Speech
  Language Pathology
University of Toronto &
  Affiliated Scientist
Health Care and Outcomes Research

Toronto Western Research Institute
Canada

Sharynne McLeod
Professor
School of Teacher Education
Charles Sturt University
Australia

Claire Penn
Professor and Chair
Department of Speech Pathology and
 Audiology
University of the Witwatersrand
South Africa

Caroline Pickstone
Honorary Research Fellow
University of Sheffield
UK

Sue Roulstone
Professor of Speech and Language
 Therapy
Faculty of Health and Life Sciences
University of the West of England
Bristol
UK

Deborah Theodoros
Professor and Head
Division of Speech Pathology &
 Co-Director

Telerehabilitation Research Unit
University of Queensland
Australia

Travis T. Threats
Professor and Chair
Department of Communication
 Sciences and Disorders
Saint Louis University
USA

Leanne Togher
Senior Research Fellow
National Health and Medical Research
 Council
Faculty of Health Sciences
The University of Sydney
Australia

Lyn Turkstra
Associate Professor
Department of Communicative
 Disorders
University of Wisconsin-Madison
USA

Sandra Van Dort
Senior Lecturer
Department of Audiology and Speech
 Sciences
Faculty of Allied Health Sciences
Universiti Kebangsaan Malaysia

Foreword by David Seedhouse

I like this book because it conveys the everyday reality of ethical decision-making as experienced by patients and practitioners, and bravely refuses to collude with the prevailing cult of bioethics.

The authors ask a central question:

> What does it mean to practise ethically? Does it mean to follow the code of ethics of one's professional association? . . . Or does it mean to embed ethical thinking into our thought processes, our attitudes, our language and our interactions?

They tell us:

> Codes of ethics can provide a context for ethical thinking and a sign that a profession is at least aware of the importance of ethics. . . . But these are not – and will never be – enough. We need to learn to 'think and act ethically in ways that are deeply embedded in routine practice'.

They are kind enough to acknowledge my own work at this point, so I'd like to reciprocate with a few words about just why their advice is so important.

Over the past 30 years or so, the 'bioethics movement' has voraciously attempted to make ethics a specialism in which only 'experts' have sufficient knowledge to decide what is ultimately ethical. In an attempt to make this bizarre claim appear plausible, most bioethicists want us to believe that ethics can be objective knowledge, and that codes of ethics, rules and protocols designed by bioethicists can and should provide intelligent ethical guidance to professionals. Many of them also insist that knowing and applying 'four principles' is pretty much all you need to be ethical.

These 'four principles' are:

- Respect for autonomy (a norm of respecting and supporting autonomous decisions)
- Nonmaleficence (a norm of avoiding the causation of harm)
- Beneficence (a group of norms pertaining to relieving, lessening, or preventing harm and providing benefits and balancing benefits against risks and costs)
- Justice (a group of norms for fairly distributing benefits, risks, and costs)

(Beauchamp and Childress, 2009)

Like many other bioethicists, Raanan Gillon, past editor of the *Journal of Medical Ethics*, seems to believe in miracles:

> *In brief, the four principles . . . approach claims that whatever your personal philosophy, politics, religion, moral theory or life stance, you will find no difficulty in committing yourself to four prima facie moral principles plus a concern for their scope of application . . . these . . . can be seen to encompass most if not all of the moral issues that arise in health care . . . 'Prima facie' . . . means that the principle is binding unless it conflicts with another moral principles – if it does then you have to choose between them. The . . . principles . . . approach provide(s) . . . a common set of moral commitments, a common moral language, and a common set of moral issues to be considered in particular cases . . . ' (p. xxii) (Gillon, 1994)*

You might just as well advance a single principle: 'Be moral' and expect everyone magically to understand and share your own moral outlook. Careful thought about ANY real life situation shows that selecting one or more of four very general principles is unlikely to provide an adequate solution, and infinitely less likely to seem 'binding' on anyone. By definition, in any heterogeneous social context, such vague principles cannot possibly provide a 'common set of moral commitments'.

The meaning of ANY code, rule, or protocol will always be in some way contradictory where protagonists have different values and priorities. Such simplicities are useful only in so far as thumbing through a store's furniture catalogue is useful: maybe some of the stuff looks good but on reflection you can't see it fitting your living room.

And that is why it is so good to read this book. Focusing on real life cases and problems can help health care workers see ethics in proper perspective:

> *'We have . . . tried to avoid basing the scenarios on one neat ethical dilemma each. Instead they are as messy as we could get them . . .'*

We swim in a sea of ethical processes in which there are no objectively right answers to be found. No matter how quasi-legal codes of ethics appear, and no matter how many 'ethics experts' tell us we should agree with their 'ethical truths', all we have in reality is ourselves, the situations we are currently in, and the ideals and behaviours we personally choose to commit to.

Every scenario in the book shows this to be true. There are no tidy answers to the husband's request that the decision to halt treatment for his wife's aphasia should be reversed (Chapter 5); just as there will always be controversy about the relationship between reducing waiting lists and discharging mobile patients who might continue to benefit from hospital care (Chapter 3).

By placing intelligent, reality-based reflection at the heart of ethical practice in speech and language therapy, the authors do an enormous service both to the profession and its patients. They also offer a beacon of light to other caring practitioners baffled and frustrated by the mystification of their practice by the self-serving bioethics industry.

Beauchamp, T., & Childress, J. (2009). *Principles of biomedical ethics* (6th ed.). Oxford: Oxford University Press.

Gillon, R. (ed) (1994). *Principles of Health Care Ethics*, Chichester: Wiley

David Seedhouse
CEO, Values Exchange (www.values-exchange.com)
Professor, AUT University, New Zealand
Professor, Staffordshire University, UK

Preface

This book on ethical issues in speech and language therapy has been immensely enjoyable to write but has, not surprisingly, presented us with some challenges. Most of these will become apparent in the book itself. Here we describe our approach – and the consequences of that approach – to the clinical scenarios we have written. In addition, we discuss the issues of international terminology, service user terminology and the service user perspective.

It is uncontroversial to assert that the field of healthcare in general is a rich breeding ground for questions of ethics. Unethical behaviour is a concept familiar to most people, even if its exact specifications are unclear. Indeed, as we shall discuss later, the concept itself is of limited use. Nevertheless, the existence of the term does suggest that a line can be drawn between actions that are in some way unethical and those that are ethical (or perhaps ethically negative and ethically positive). Most importantly, it underlines the fact that questions of ethics are of central concern to users and suppliers of health services, i.e. everyone.

As will be obvious to anyone who has perused any of the literature on healthcare ethics, the vast majority has been written either by doctors or by (medical) ethicists writing about doctors. There is a corresponding literature in speech and language therapy, but to date it is a field that has seen only limited development. We argue in Chapter 1 that it is not going to be productive to wait for further development to come from doctors or, at this stage, (medical) ethicists. Therefore, this book is intended to contribute to the developing foundation of a field of ethics in speech and language therapy. There is a slight danger in this of being perceived as part of an indiscriminate overdevelopment of ethics (what Fulford, Dickenson and Murray (2002) call 'ethics with everything' (p. 1)) but the response from therapists to the news that the book was being written has suggested that the discipline is some considerable distance from such a situation.

The book is written in the first instance for speech and language therapists involved or interested in clinical practice. This includes clinicians, managers (who may or may not have direct clinical contact) and people working in a support capacity (speech and language therapy assistants, in UK parlance). The book is also intended to be for students currently on speech and language therapy courses and those providing the education. We hope that in this capacity the book will stimulate discussion and development to help prepare students for the ethically rich world that awaits them.

For entirely practical reasons the book is based on clinical practice in English-speaking countries (or in some cases where English may be one of many languages spoken) and is aimed at a readership in those countries. Readers from other countries with an interest in speech and language therapy are more than welcome to join us.

Although the book has been written with an audience from speech and language therapy in mind, we hope that other health professionals will take the opportunity to browse some of the issues. During the course of writing the book we have learned a lot from a disparate range of healthcare ethics sources, most notably the voluminous ethics literature arising from medicine but also the smaller and equally stimulating literature from nursing and the other allied health professions. In fact, one of our main aims has been to facilitate access to this broad literature for readers who might otherwise not happen upon it. In many cases our learning has taken the form of 'We have that issue as well' or 'Perhaps our profession should be discussing that issue'. It would be nice to think that some other health professionals might experience that reaction on reading about ethics and speech and language therapy.

Much of the discussion of ethics as it relates directly to clinical practice is based around clinical scenarios representing a variety of aspects of speech and language therapy practice. The potential benefits of using case examples or clinical scenarios are demonstrated by their widespread use in many areas of both healthcare and ethics literature. They offer a means of populating a book with people and issues that are familiar to readers, thereby increasing readers' sense of involvement. But often this is not what happens. In our experience, scenarios are often very brief and are almost always written in the third person from the perspective of a detached observer, complete with a narrator's infallible ability to simplify complex issues. In clinical life, ethical issues are not generally presented to us on such a clean plate. The fact that there is some ethical issue to be considered makes itself known to us in a multitude of unpredictable ways: a stray phrase overheard in conversation or leaping out from an e-mail alerts us to the need to pay ethical attention; a sense of psychological unease refuses to go away until we work out what is bothering us; a night of interrupted sleep reminds us that we have not finished wondering what to say to a patient first thing tomorrow morning. While it is neither possible nor entirely desirable to avoid a third-person description of situations that challenge our ethical thinking, we have tried to include some of the sense of introspection, inference and sometimes incompleteness that characterises ethical thought. We have done this by means of a variety of narrative techniques: the thoughts of a man with a rapidly deteriorating neurological condition; a series of overlapping e-mails between two newly qualified therapists, and between a patient and his son; a letter of complaint from a patient's husband – the sort of letter that drops on your desk and changes your day. We have also tried to avoid basing the scenarios on one neat ethical dilemma each. Instead they are as messy as we could get them without sacrificing clarity of information. This, at least, has been our intention. At this point we should add that all the characters in the scenarios are entirely the product of our imagination. Elsewhere in the book we have used pseudonyms for people featuring in descriptions of our own clinical experience.

Once we had written these scenarios we presented a variety of clinically experienced commentators with the task of discerning and discussing the issues either contained in or provoked by them. In line with our approach to the style of the scenarios, we did not ask commentators to propose 'correct' ethical courses of action, though in some cases these seem to have arisen naturally. Instead, we tried to facilitate the expression of the variety of perspectives that is characteristic of clinical life.

The scenario commentaries have come from various countries where English is (one of) the first language(s). The underlying shared language has been accompanied by a wide variation in regional flavours of vocabulary and phraseology. We have thus been faced with a choice of international terms. In the majority of the book, we have chosen to use the terms 'speech and language therapy' and 'speech and language therapist' (the latter abbreviated to SLT as appropriate) on the sole grounds that the book is published in the United Kingdom. In the commentaries, however, we have kept to the term of choice of the commentator (e.g. speech-language pathologist). Here we have also left unaltered other terms (e.g. Bed #2, practicum) and spellings (behavior, realize) that are not standard in the United Kingdom, except where a change to a more general term appeared to be needed to avoid misunderstanding.

Issues of terminology can, of course, have more serious implications than whether individual words reflect local or international usage. For example, Wright-St Clair and Seedhouse (2005) highlight the significant message that can be conveyed by a seemingly subtle change in emphasis, such as by rephrasing 'client-centred practice' – an apparently noble aim at first glance – as 'person-centred practice'. Accordingly, we have had to consider the terms used to describe the people who use speech and language therapy services. 'Patient' is the most established term in health services around the world but is recognised as having arisen from a medical model of healthcare. 'Client' is another term in fairly widespread use, though with possible connotations (not inherently good or bad) of a business relationship and without any emphasis on individual personhood. 'Service user' has become more widespread as social models of empowerment and inclusion have developed, though, like any two-word term in competition with single words, it can feel slightly cumbersome. Other potential multiword terms such as 'person using speech and language therapy services' (along the lines of 'person with aphasia' [see below]) were also felt to be unwieldy. We have addressed the challenge of which word to use mainly by using whichever term felt most appropriate in the context.

The issue of single and multiword terms is also a challenge in relation to the way in which we refer to communication disorders (or indeed impairments or difficulties) and the people who live with them. In general, we have tried to use terminology which both differentiates between individuals and their communication and places the people themselves centre-stage (see Folkins [1992] on the website of the American Speech-Language-Hearing Association for useful guidance on these issues). For example, the term 'aphasic' is no longer in any way acceptable (if indeed it ever was) as a stand-alone noun applied to a person who has aphasia. Perhaps even less acceptable is the use of a disease or trauma process to label people (e.g. 'TBIs tend to . . .'). The use of 'aphasic' as a modifying adjective (e.g. 'a 50-year old aphasic man') is likely to be heading in a similar direction. Multiword terms (e.g. 'a person who has/is living with aphasia) tend to convey a greater sense of respect for the person and to recognise the separation between the individual and the communication disorder. As with the term 'service user', multiword terms relating to communication disorders can be similarly cumbersome, which itself risks damaging the status and recognition of the disorder (and resources allocated to it). We have tried to steer a sensitive path between these two positions.

Obviously, one way to solve the dilemma over terminology would be to ask the people who experience the communication disorder/impairment/difficulty for their views, though any assumption that there might be agreement is perhaps naive. This approach to inclusion has significant ethical implications which feature widely in the book, and it brings us to the linked, and rather more weighty, issue of the service user perspective in general. We have sought views on the various ethical issues in the book from a variety of professionals and spent a considerable amount of time pondering the desirability and practicality of including service users as well. In the end practicality won, since we felt we could not do justice in a single book to the broad selection of views required for true representativeness. Our intention is to revisit the issues raised by the scenarios in a separate work based on contributions from service users.

Acknowledgements

This book represents a synthesis of conversations held over many years with speech and language therapy clients, and with a variety of speech and language therapy colleagues and other health professionals far too numerous to list individually. We hope that the content of the book will stand as acknowledgement of the significant contribution made by all these people.

In addition we would like to thank the following people for their contributions: Liz Barnett, Veronica Goddard, Alice Owen, Caroline Pickstone and Sue Pownall for helpful discussions (though responsibility for the opinions in the book rests with the authors). Special thanks go to Maggie Campbell and Joan Rosenthal for their perceptive comments on the text and once more to Maggie Campbell for her support throughout the project. Lindy would also like to thank Archie for ensuring that she took regular time away from the computer to go for a walk.

Finally we would like to express our gratitude to the various colleagues who agreed (with encouraging enthusiasm) to write commentaries for the book.

1 Introduction

This book is about healthcare ethics relevant to speech and language therapists. In it we aim not just to deal with the dramas and dilemmas which tend to characterise thinking on ethics – the 'Should I do A or B?' ethics – but also to delve into the subtleties of attempting to understand people with communication disorders well enough to represent them, of managing interactions in a way that affirms and empowers people, and of making fair decisions about resource allocation.

The primary aim of the book is for debate into ethical issues to be stimulated within the profession of speech and language therapy, prompted by description of various clinical scenarios. Equally importantly, the book is concerned with highlighting the need to consider ethical issues in all aspects of our clinical practice. While we will need to invoke a number of concepts from moral philosophy, the book is primarily about clinical work and the ethical issues experienced by clinicians. It is written by two clinicians with an interest in the relationship between healthcare and ethics.

Ethics is basically about people and how they relate to each other. So rather than starting with discussion of exact definitions of ethics, different approaches to healthcare ethics or the relationship between ethics and, say, law, we are instead going to consider some examples of the impact of ethical issues on therapists and therapeutic interactions. We start with a speech and language therapist, Alison, who is mulling over a problem in the small hours – a familiar experience for people working in healthcare.

The basic problem is that if I ask her, she might say no. On the one hand Rebecca's mum hasn't said I *can't* pass information to the rest of the team. On the other hand, she doesn't actually know I know anything about Rebecca's dad. I think Rebecca would have a much better chance of settling into school if they knew her father was in jail. What was it Rebecca had said? 'He did a bank.' From a preschool child! It sounded like he was violent towards his family before he went to jail as well. It might help the school to understand why Rebecca was so timid and not quite ready for the classroom. But she has to go to school next year and this is the only school in town. I want her to have a good first year; her future depends on it.

Alison rarely lost sleep over her work, but this case was worrying her. She almost wished little Rebecca hadn't told her about her father. Alison had been seeing Rebecca for blocks of therapy on and off for most of the year. Rebecca had been so timid and with such delayed speech and language at the start of the year that she hardly said a thing. But as the year passed and her communication skills progressed, Rebecca had warmed to Alison and started to tell her more and more about preschool, her friends, pets and siblings. One day when her mother was unable to join in the session because of a medical appointment, Rebecca told Alison about her father. She was quite tearful and said she hoped he wouldn't be coming home for Christmas.

Now Alison was worrying about whether to pass on this information. The team's psychologist was due to assess Rebecca the following week to provide a report to the local school about Rebecca's school-readiness and support needs. Rebecca's mother had not said 'no' to sharing that information, but Alison felt that it might make the difference between success and failure for Rebecca in her first year of school.

The dilemma at the heart of this scenario is typical of a traditional view of ethics – Alison has a choice of X or Y and she must choose one of them. Basically, she is faced with the option to divulge the information (and risk damaging the relationship with the mother) or not to divulge the information (and risk undermining the contribution of the psychologist to Rebecca's future and potentially risk aspects of Rebecca's future itself). There are various more subtle options – for example, Alison could attempt to negotiate the release of information with the mother – but at its heart the decision is 'to divulge or not to divulge'.

The focus on dilemmas, we argue, constrains understanding of ethical practice. We would like to illustrate a wider perspective by standing back temporarily from the world of speech and language therapy. In their research paper entitled 'Saying no to the staff', Finlay, Antaki and Walton (2008) describe in detail what at first sight appear to be a fairly routine set of interactions in a home for people with intellectual disability. The residents have high support needs and most have only a small number of intelligible words at their disposal. The authors provide a context for the article by highlighting the fact that care staff have to negotiate a course between two potentially contradictory obligations. The first is the obligation to respect the preferences and decisions of the residents (and, by implication, to find some way of establishing what these preferences and decisions are). The second, seemingly more mundane obligation is to monitor residents' weight regularly as part of general health screening. The article describes in detail the interactions between care staff and Matthew, who is known to be averse to stepping onto the scales to be weighed, but who expresses himself primarily via nonverbal vocalisation. The analysis of attempts by a member of staff to persuade Matthew to step onto the scales (while somehow respecting his preference not to) illustrates the subtlety of approach that is required.

An initial request (or perhaps invitation) by the member of staff – Jill – is worded as 'Dy'wanna get weighed?', to which Matthew responds with a vocalisation that is interpreted as a refusal. Jill then issues a second invitation ('Dy'wanna nother go?')

and then, following a second refusal, a third ('Shall we get weighed?'). The authors analyse the wording of Jill's contributions and her selection of particular phrases from a potentially large set of eligible phrases. They describe the second invitation as a 'no-blame formulation' in that the reference to 'another go' – even though there hasn't really been a first one – serves to absolve Matthew of blame for his inaction. They also highlight the collective phrasing of the third attempt as signalling a task that Jill and Matthew are to accomplish together. In fact, after various contributions to the interaction from other staff, Matthew wins this particular battle of wills and leaves the room without being weighed.

The linguistic sensitivity with which these negotiations are undertaken should be entirely familiar to clinicians working in the field of communication disorder. What the authors illustrate in particular is the link between the words that make their way to the conversational surface and the ethical issues lying much deeper, in this case active respect for Matthew's choice and the contradictory obligation to care for his health needs. The following extract, worth quoting in full, illustrates what important work is going on in these interactions:

> Choice and control are issues that arise in the way people talk to each other, in which utterances are taken up and which are ignored, in how and what options are offered, in how preferences are expressed, how information is presented, how spaces are opened up for people to express preference and how spaces are shut down. (Finlay et al., 2008, p. 56)

The authors stress the importance of being able to express such preferences for people with communication difficulties, who may have limited opportunities to exercise control over other aspects of their lives.

In the circumstances described above it is unlikely that Jill would be seen as facing an ethical dilemma in her choice of words, yet there are serious ethical considerations involved. Language here *is* the surface manifestation of ethics. We explore this view further in a second scenario.

This example is from my (RB) clinical practice. Although it seems like a relatively minor incident, it has stayed with me for over 20 years. I was in my fourth year of clinical practice, my first as a specialist in neurology. I was feeling rather pleased with myself. Specialist status meant – surely had to mean – that I had particular expertise and could therefore contribute more. I felt established, useful and important, a pleasing combination.

Although I had been involved in the assessment and management of people with motor neurone disease (MND) on acute hospital wards, I had worked with only one man from the time of his diagnosis to his death. I had tried to help him make the most of a communication aid, given rather inexpert advice on managing his increasing difficulty with swallowing (this being before dysphagia management came of age) and visited him in the hospice. For most of this time I had worried about being asked questions I couldn't answer, but I had also found it a moving and positive experience.

I was now working with my second person with MND. Mrs Davies had known of her diagnosis for almost a year and was becoming increasingly restricted to the house, not because of her mobility but because of the difficulty in making herself understood. I had introduced the possibility of trying a communication aid and she had reluctantly agreed at least to look at it.

I collected a potentially suitable electronic aid and drove out to Mrs Davies's house on a stuffy summer's afternoon. Her daughter had not been able to come to this appointment but had said she was happy for it to go ahead. Mrs Davies opened the front door and led me into the front room. It was oppressively hot and the quietness outside seemed to make the situation quite tense. We exchanged a couple of phrases about the weather and then I found myself asking how her speech had been, thinking as I said it, 'I *know* how her speech must have been. I can hear it.' Still, this was my job; this was what I was getting paid to ask for detail about. And then, seemingly equally as inadvertently, I asked, 'Have you had any problems with your swallowing yet?' She gave a long, drawn out, dysarthric wail and, almost out of breath, half-whispered, 'Please don't say *yet*.'

I found myself simultaneously registering the clarity of her articulation and realising the momentous implications of such a short and apparently innocuous word. Mrs Davies was inconsolable for the next 10 minutes and the communication aid had clearly become an irrelevance. Eventually she succeeded in gathering herself and offered me a cup of tea. We managed a few minutes of superficial, calming conversation and then both agreed that the session would be better reconvened for another day. I headed out to the car feeling flat and a bit helpless. I imagined Mrs Davies sitting in her room looking at the blank television for a while.

This event clearly does not constitute an ethical dilemma. I did not ponder whether one course of action would be better than another. In fact the question left my head so quickly there would not have been time to contemplate it anyway. It would be a harsh judge who would interpret this interaction in terms of 'unethical conduct'. It was not even possible to say with any certainty that it was a 'bad thing' in itself – Mrs Davies might in some way have gained some benefit from the catharsis. And yet, in this context and at this time, the word 'yet' had caused her acute psychological distress and I felt that I had caused that distress by being thoughtless. And that was exactly the point – I had not necessarily chosen the wrong phrase but I had not considered the implications of the phrase that I did use.

Thinking about it afterwards, I was struck by the thought that there is an ethical dimension to the choice of single words, phrases, intonations. They have implications for their recipients, often acutely sensitised by the vulnerability of their circumstances. I felt sad and I am quite sure Mrs Davies felt despondent. It is not always possible, or even desirable, to avoid saying things that make people sad, but in this case the use of the word 'yet' was insensitive and I could have broached the subject in a way that was less distressing.

Like the interactions described in Finlay et al.'s residential home article, this last clinical scenario is a long way from what could be termed a dilemma. Nor does it feel like an entirely 'clinical' issue. It involves, at its heart, the effects of an action that happens to be speech.

Speech acts are a well-known phenomenon in the study of pragmatics and they are thus familiar territory (at least in a theoretical sense) for speech and language therapists (SLTs). Savulescu, Foddy and Rogers (2006), writing in the *Journal of Medical Ethics*, make the important link between speech acts and ethical theory in relation to the words we choose in talking to people who are dealing with a health problem of one sort or another: 'When we say something to a person who is suffering, we perform a speech act that can have significant impact on their wellbeing. It is morally important why we say what we say' (p. 8).

This focus on the subtleties of language should not be taken to imply that ethical dilemmas do not occur in speech and language therapy. Although as a profession we do not tend to deal with what are variously called 'neon' ethics (Braunack-Mayer, 2001), 'science fiction' ethics (Cribb & Duncan, 2002) and even 'gee-whizz' ethics (Fulford et al., 2002) – the headline news, life-and-death, sometimes legally mediated decisions that make their way into public consciousness – we are certainly faced with choices about the best way to act. Indeed, many of the later scenarios in the book incorporate decisions to be pondered by SLTs. But focusing on ethical dilemmas distracts attention from the fact that healthcare is fundamentally an ethical business. As Parker and Dickenson (2001) put it, 'the danger of this concentration on crises is that it creates the impression that medicine and healthcare is otherwise unproblematic' (p. 125). We would go further and say that ethics is not just about problems but also about attitudes and the underlying direction of health work.

The situations involving Alison, the residential home staff and Mrs Davies serve to illustrate different aspects of healthcare ethics to which we return later in the book. We now step back temporarily from the direct focus on people attempting to negotiate an ethically positive route through their daily work to consider some of the ethical landscape in the background.

What is ethics?

Ethics is often equated with decisions of high moral magnitude and associated with weighty concepts of right and wrong or good and evil. The relevance of ethics to the daily experience of working in healthcare is not always easy to perceive. A definition proposed by Seedhouse (1998) highlights this daily relevance. He refers to ethics as 'a process of deliberation about how best to act in the presence of other lives' (p. 47). This definition may better characterise our thoughts on the way to work, or indeed, as many people will have experienced, in the middle of a sleepless night: how are we going to help X achieve something? how are we going to guide Y away from doing something else? which should we do first?

Why is ethics important?

Many writers have highlighted the centrality of health to our lives. To quote Seedhouse (2002a) again, 'all health care practice takes place in the ethical realm' (p. 253). However, to a large extent this sound moral foundation to healthcare is taken for granted. During training as health professionals we devote large amounts of our time and effort to the assimilation of theoretical and technical knowledge together with professional and clinical skills. Relatively speaking, we devote only very small amounts of time and effort to consideration of the huge ethical implications of what we are learning to do. The knowledge and skills we learn in training (and develop throughout our careers) are what Sim (1997) terms the *means* of providing healthcare. They form the focus of much of our thinking and discussion as health professionals. Ethics, on the other hand, provides a way of thinking about the proper '*ends*' of healthcare (Sim, 1997) – the whole point of all that time spent learning and refining the means. It may be the case that in their broadest sense the ultimate ends of healthcare remain relatively stable, i.e. the optimisation of everyone's health potential, but the subgoals shift as society develops and courses of action influence each other, such that decisions over what to do and how to act have to be taken within a dynamic, shifting ethical environment. And of course the major contribution to the dynamic, shifting ethical environment that constitutes healthcare comes from people – service users, carers, clinical staff, domestic staff, managers and many more. This is a fundamentally human endeavour, bursting with other people's lives.

The development of new technologies and approaches to healthcare often serves to alert the public to questions about whether such technologies *should* be put into practice simply because they *can* be. Medical issues most commonly perform this alerting function, but related questions can be asked of all aspects of healthcare. Does this therapy programme actually work? Is it an approach my client prefers? Will it benefit my client? Is it worth a try even if we don't know whether it works? Is it cost effective for my employer? Who should receive the therapy? Who could we be seeing instead? What impact does my instigation of this therapy have on service delivery by my colleagues? It is easy to conceptualise these questions as purely clinical in nature, involving clinical decision making, but it is fundamentally impossible to take a clinical decision that does not have ethical implications one way or another.

We can illustrate this point with an example from a recent teaching discussion (RB) of ethics in cleft lip and palate, during which a student raised the issue of how, and particularly *when*, to bring to the notice of parents a suspicion that their child might have some further serious condition as well as the cleft. Another student then queried whether this was an ethical issue or a clinical one. The clinical considerations to this question loom large. You would want to be sure of your clinical ground but not want to delay any opportunity for more detailed assessment and intervention. You would need to consider the clinical roles within your team and judge who should follow up your clinical hunch. Importantly, though, your handy textbook on clinical decision making in cleft palate may not address this issue at all – since it is a byproduct of the central clinical issue – and it is especially unlikely to deal with the sense of conflicting obligations you feel to the child, the parents and your team. You don't want to give them the wrong information, but you might have to put them through some anxiety in order to find out one way or another. The clinical and ethical aspects of this situation represent two sides of the same coin.

There is also a sense in which, as we shall see in the following section, recognition of the importance of ethics is of particular significance in the field of communication disorder. Communication is one of the most sensitive expressions of 'acting in the presence of other lives', and the essence of our work as SLTs is about helping people who have a specific difficulty in affecting others' lives through communication and giving expression to how they want others to act in the presence of their own lives. SLTs spend their working lives in psychologically intimate relationships with people who are at some sort of disadvantage in their dealings with others.

We now consider the recent expansion in literature on the subject of healthcare ethics and the extent to which this literature is applicable to speech and language therapy or informs its practice.

Healthcare ethics literature

Ethics in medicine (usually termed either medical ethics or bioethics) has now reached sufficient critical mass to be considered a discipline in its own right, as evidenced by the proliferation of journals dedicated to the subject, such as the *Journal of Medical Ethics*, *Cambridge Quarterly of Healthcare Ethics* and *Journal of Clinical Ethics*. Related fields have also made a start in this direction, for example the journal *Nursing Ethics*.

Clearly, there are areas of medicine and medical ethics that are not essentially relevant to speech and language therapy practice. Most SLTs will have no professional involvement in decisions about termination of pregnancy, except perhaps where their clients are having to ponder the decision themselves. Other hot topics in medical care, such as genetic testing and disclosure of information on transmissible diseases, are outside the areas where SLTs generally practise. On the other hand, many of the insights provided by the general debates in medical ethics are relevant to speech and language therapy.

On a theoretical level, for example, recent articles in the *Journal of Medical Ethics* (Freeman, 2006; Sokol, 2006) have lamented the unhelpful distance between (medical) ethicists and (medical) practitioners. Sokol (2006) refers to 'abstruse theorising and ignorance of practical medicine' (p. 1226) on the part of ethicists, and Freeman (2006) says that although ethical theory may provide some guidance, it does not provide sufficient help in individual cases. While speech and language therapy is rarely, if ever, specifically subject to the pronouncements of moral philosophers, there is certainly a parallel gap between ethical theory and speech and language therapy practice. Faced with the issue of client confidentiality at the opening of this chapter, Alison is unlikely to turn to one of the major medical ethics textbooks to prompt her thinking, much less to Aristotle or John Stuart Mill. This is an issue to which we return later when discussing ethical decision making.

On a more concrete level, the medical ethics literature features regular debate on, for instance, rationing of services, something with which all healthcare professionals are familiar. Browne and Browne (2007) discuss ways in which clinicians sometimes violate practice guidelines (i.e. bend the rules) so that their patients can derive a benefit they might otherwise be denied (because, for example, they do not fit predefined criteria for access to treatment). They further differentiate between *offensive* violations, where most people stick to the rules and the clinician in question wants to secure an advantage for a patient, and *defensive* violations, where other people may well be breaking the rules and the clinician follows suit so as not to *dis*advantage a patient. The article may have originated in medicine, but it is not too difficult to imagine circumstances in speech and language therapy where the concepts would be relevant.

Given (a) the volume of medical ethics material available and (b) the fact that there is at least some overlap between medical ethics and the world of speech and language therapy, anyone who has read this far might be forgiven for wondering why we need to consider ethics in speech and language therapy separately. The answer, of course, is that speech and language therapy is special. Just as there are issues that arise in medical ethics but not speech and language therapy, the reverse, i.e. ethical issues that arise in speech and language therapy but not in medicine, is consistently if perhaps less transparently true.

Speech and language therapy is fundamentally about people's ability to communicate. Despite the growth of work in dysphagia, it is still communication that defines us as a profession and it is our body of knowledge concerning communication disorder that differentiates us from other professions. Seedhouse's (1998) 'how best to act in the presence of other lives' might justifiably be paraphrased by SLTs as how best to *inter*act in the presence of other lives.

A paper by Malloy et al. (2006) includes a potentially revealing comment on doctors' perceptions of communication disorder. The authors explore a model of moral intensity originally conceived by Thomas Jones (1991) as a way of delineating factors which might make an ethical dilemma more intense. One of the factors identified is proximity, defined as the relative physical, social or psychological closeness between decision-maker and patient. The authors exemplify this construct as follows: 'A physician who is able to communicate verbally with a patient will have a greater sense of proximity than will a physician attending to a patient with severe cognitive impairment and inability to communicate verbally' (Malloy et al., 2006, p. 286). It is likely that anyone – SLT or physician – who has experienced the intense interactions that can occur with people whose communication is severely restricted might take issue with the somewhat unidimensional view expressed in this statement. At the very least, it suggests that it is not enough for the speech and language therapy profession to rely on the field of medical ethics for exploration of the ethical issues arising from communication disorder. An alternative perspective can be found in a study of dementia care by Brannelly (2006) in which observers noted consistency of what was termed 'social regard' by practitioners (care staff, social workers, etc.) interacting with people with dementia. This consistency was not necessarily a positive thing in its own right since some of the practitioners consistently approached people with dementia with social regard and others consistently did not. The important factor is that this consistency was applied 'regardless of [the person with dementia's] ability or communicative capacity' (Brannelly, 2006, p. 203).

Disruption of people's ability to communicate thoughts and feelings takes us deep into people's lives and presents us as therapists with the responsibility of handling a world of ethical subtleties in a sensitive way. It also highlights the possibility of viewing communication as a basic human right alongside health, food and shelter (Horner Catt, 2000) (an issue we return to in Chapter 8). A few examples by way of illustration:

▩ An intellectually disabled man has always expressed a fear of illness and is now terminally ill. Someone needs to assess the extent to which he can understand what is going to happen to him and to balance his right to know with his capacity for dealing with and communicating distress.

▩ The family of a five-year-old girl who has had repair of a unilateral cleft lip and palate is offered a series of speech and language therapy appointments. They attend one but then stop responding to contact. The girl is at a critical point in her emotional and social development and yet the family appears to have made an autonomous decision not to attend for therapy. How far can the SLT pursue this? Is it really the SLT's decision? Is the only course of action to wait until she reaches adulthood? And then do what?

▩ Demands on funding mean that a Stroke Group needs to be closed down, as a result of which an aphasic woman, whose husband has recently died, finds her access to social interaction all but curtailed. Her language problems make it difficult for her to make use of standard services or to meet people without help, and the Stroke Group has until now provided the only regular time when the skill of the therapist and the supportive enthusiasm of the other participants made communication less effortful than it generally is. Her language is not likely to improve and other clients have more obviously pressing needs.

The therapy relationship between clients and SLTs often develops over significant periods of time, with many hours spent together in highly charged interactions. Picture a 13-year-old stutterer – bullied at school, sullen and resentful – in her first session with a speech and language therapist who her mother has finally persuaded her to see. She is probably hoping for a rapid, responsibility-free cure – anything less and she would have been right not to listen to her mother all along. For the therapist the first job is to establish some sort of relationship that can be prolonged. But prolonged to where? Improvement? Control? Awareness? Acceptance? Despair? The therapist might be persuading the girl to engage in therapy only for her to experience the crushing realisation that this speech pattern is never going to disappear completely. On the other hand, the SLT might see someone developing into a self-confident and competent young woman who is so free of the pressures of dysfluency that both of them have difficulty recalling the person she once was.

And just below the surface of the desire for a cure lie other unspoken hopes: of being able to talk to someone about what it's like; of being able to talk to someone who knows something about the subject; of dealing with someone who will be honest with you but who can judge the best time to give difficult information; of having someone on your side, someone who will fight your corner, someone who will get you out of the mire at school; of working with someone who will put themselves out for you.

This combination of a communication disorder and the relationships involved in trying to manage it is unique. As such, it raises unique ethical issues requiring dedicated (in both senses of the word) discussion.

Another reason to conclude that speech and language therapy requires its own literature on clinical ethics is that even where the issues discussed in medical ethics journals overlap with speech and language therapy, the discussion itself takes place, in effect, out of sight of the profession. Theoretically we could all browse medical ethics books and journals and interpret what we find there for our own purposes. Realistically it is going to be a very determined SLT who takes time away from clinical work to check out medical ethics literature on the off-chance that something will resonate with speech and language therapy practice.

It is important to acknowledge that this book is a contribution to a small but growing literature on ethics in speech and language therapy. By way of example there are Irwin, Pannbacker, Powell and Vekovius's *Ethics for Speech-Language Pathologists and Audiologists* (2007); a special issue of *Seminars in Speech and Language* (2003, 24[4]); Hersh's work on discharge in aphasia (Hersh, 2002, 2003) (to which we return in Chapter 5); various discussions of the ethical aspects of dysphagia, particularly non-oral feeding (Landes, 1999; Sharp & Bryant, 2003; Sharp & Genesen, 1996); and Kenny, Lincoln and Balandin's (2007) recent speech and language therapy incursion into the *Journal of Medical Ethics*. In addition, more closely centred within speech and language therapy professional circles there have been a number of discussions on websites and/or articles in professional publications. Other examples include the *ASHA Leader Online*, part of the website of the American Speech-Language-Hearing Association (ASHA), which features short discussions and statements on ethical topics (e.g. statements on cultural competence [ASHA, 2005]) and client abandonment [ASHA, 2008b]), and the professional bulletin of Speech Pathology Australia (*ACQuiring Knowledge in Speech, Language and Hearing* or 'ACQ'), which also has occasional articles on ethics (e.g. R. Cross, Leitão & McAllister, 2008).

This might look like a fair amount of discussion on the subject of ethics when gathered into one paragraph. However, given the breadth of clinical practice and the number of professionals and service users involved worldwide, the material is actually spread pretty thin and is dissipated across various forums, some more widely accessible than others (the *ASHA Leader Online*, for example, is open to public view). From our point of view the profession currently needs as much in the way of ethics debate as it can get.

Morality, values, law and ethics

Having established that ethics in speech and language therapy is worthy of discussion, we now introduce some concepts associated with ethics. The relationships between concepts such as morality, law and ethics are described in detail by various authors (e.g. Hendrick, 2000; Sim, 1997), and we do not intend to add detailed discussion here. However, a brief overview is warranted in the interests of starting from a reasonably firm conceptual foundation.

Ethics and morality

For SLTs considering whether to divulge possibly confidential information to a colleague, the relationship between the philosophical concepts of ethics and morality may seem to be of little interest and certainly of no practical use for the task at hand. This, largely, is the line followed in this book, in part because various authors on healthcare ethics describe the two concepts, in some senses at least, as effectively interchangeable (Horner Catt, 2000; Malloy et al., 2006). This does not mean to say, however, that distinctions are not drawn between the two concepts. In fact, these same authors highlight possible distinctions: Horner Catt (2000) refers to a delineation between social good in general (morality) and individual good (ethics), and Malloy et al. (2006) (following Aristotle) describe morals as 'universal concepts that transcend cultural variation and practice' and ethics as 'principles particular to context' (p. 286). Likewise, Sim (1997) states that while there is no real difference between 'ethical' and 'moral' in some uses of the terms, there is a sense in which ethical is taken to refer to a 'specific code of moral behaviour associated with a particular professional role' (p. 12). So one interpretation is that the relationship between ethics and morality can be conceptualised as the former being a systematisation of the latter. Indeed, Colicutt McGrath (2007) describes ethics as the systematic study of moral values, in the course of which those values are translated into standards and rules of personal and cultural practices.

From our perspective, it is important to establish that although ethical standards and rules might arise from the systematic study of morality (and in their turn give rise to statements or codes of ethics), we would not want to equate ethics with rules or codes. This point is relevant to some of the commentaries later in the book, because in some formulations (e.g. Downie & Macnaughton, 2007) the concept of (professional) ethics is largely interpreted in terms of its regulatory function. Moreover, in some parts of the world (notably the USA) the term 'ethics' relates primarily to rules (of conduct) and codes (of ethics), leaving wider areas of debate to come under the heading of 'morality'.

For us, and for our view of the daily practice of speech and language therapy, ethics and morality *are* functionally interchangeable, relating as they do to 'choices large and small that impact others – sometimes to enhance others' lives and sometimes to harm them' (Horner Catt, 2000, p. 138), though Horner Catt herself applies this phrase only to morality. As we discuss in Chapter 2, a wider view of ethics has significant implications in terms of recognising the limitations of codes of ethics for addressing the issues that arise in clinical practice, some of which are described in the scenarios.

Ethics and law

Although there are laws covering a huge variety of behaviours – for example, the UK has a 1969 law prohibiting the tattooing of people under 18 (other than by a medical practitioner) regardless of parental consent – it is also not difficult to imagine situations in professional work about which the law would have little or nothing to say. The decision (outlined above) to stop running a Stroke Group, for example, is very unlikely to be the subject of legal debate. The fact that the decision has ethical implications, on the other hand – whether it is the right or wrong thing to do in the light of other service needs – is less debatable, though this may not makes the decision itself any clearer.

It is, of course, the case that a variety of laws *are* entirely relevant to SLTs in their work, such as laws concerned with the rights of children and with anti-discrimination legislation. A key point here, as outlined by Sim (1997), is that the law works in terms of minimum standards below which behaviour should not fall. This is not to say that everyone agrees on the ethical rightness or wrongness of the area *below* the minimum legal standard. In other words, some people may think that a law is not ethically acceptable. Above these minimum standards there is significant scope for ethically good or bad decision making. We will take another example from my (RB) early – I'd like to plead inexperience – clinical practice, when I was working with a patient with dysphonia who had had nasendoscopy recommended by the Ear, Nose and Throat surgeon. She was, perhaps not surprisingly, somewhat averse to the idea of having a tube inserted up her nose and I took to persuading her of the benefits, unwittingly painting myself into a corner at the same time. The crucial point in the discussion came when I claimed that the procedure was 'not that bad', which prompted her to ask whether I had experienced it. If I said 'No', my claims would dissolve; a pause would be equivalent to an admission that I hadn't but that I was possibly contemplating some claim to the contrary; 'Yes' would be lying but might persuade her to undergo the procedure. These were the only alternatives that presented themselves in the very short space of thinking time. Perhaps some variant of 'No, but I've talked to people who have' would have offered another alternative, though at the time that would not have been strictly true either. At the risk of alienating the book's readers before we've really started, I must report that I said 'Yes', and she had the nasendoscopy done, as did I shortly afterwards in an effort to assuage my guilt. As far as I am aware I did not contravene any law (though I'll reiterate the plea of inexperience just in case), but I have had a number of debates since then with students as to whether this was an unethical action on my part. The outcome for the patient was fundamentally positive but the 'ends justifies the means' approach, although legal, seems to teeter dangerously close to the top of a slippery ethical slope and I certainly did not feel comfortable with it at the time.

Ethics and values

Cutting across ethical concepts of good, bad, right and wrong and, more importantly, the deliberation of how to act in the presence of other lives are the various
things that people value and that have to be considered in making ethical decisions.
For example, we might place value on a friendship, an heirloom, trade unions,
honesty, the fact that the shop down the road sells pomegranates, etc. The list of
our values is unlikely to be an exact match for those of even the people closest to
us, let alone all the people with whom we come into contact in our working lives.

Some of these values are more clearly relevant to our interactions with other
people's lives than others. So my valuing of the availability of pomegranates might
be ethically neutral for most other people (though the question of how they arrive
in my local shop may not). My valuing of trade unions, on the other hand, may
come into direct conflict with the views of a patient whose company is in almost
permanent dispute with its workforce. Taking this one step further, we could ask
whether, in my interaction with this patient, I am ethically obliged to help her
communicate anti-union sentiments, should that be her stated wish. Moreover, it is
not inconceivable that some areas of therapy, such as voice work with transsexual
clients, might present significant challenges in relation to the values espoused by
some therapists.

Structure of the book

Having discussed the importance of ethics to speech and language therapy, in
Chapter 2 we look at resources such as codes of ethics and ethical decision-making
frameworks and consider their role in ethical practice. The central six chapters (3–8)
are based on specific areas of clinical practice: dysphagia; intellectual and sensory
impairments; acquired communication disorders; paediatric speech and language
disorders; degenerative conditions in ageing; and, finally, service provision and
management. The selected areas cover many of the major areas in speech and language therapy, and we hope that the issues raised will be relevant outside their
area of origin. Each of the six chapters has a similar structure, incorporating two
clinical scenarios (written by us), two commentaries on each of the scenarios
(written by people who are not us) and a discussion section.

For the commentaries we have invited leading SLTs from a wide range of
countries (Australia, Canada, Malaysia, New Zealand, South Africa, the UK and
the USA) to bring their experience to bear on the issues raised by the scenarios.
The commentators were asked not to use the 'language of ethics' (e.g. beneficence,
veracity) but to discuss in plain language why they felt the scenarios presented
challenging issues. The commentators have tackled the task in different ways,
and by and large we have chosen not to interfere with this. In some cases our

discussion has picked up issues highlighted by both commentators and in others we have pulled out issues that were not the focus of either of the commentators' efforts. Guidance to the commentators also included a request not to include many references, in order to facilitate focus on the topic under discussion itself. In some instances the approach taken by an individual commentator meant that inclusion of a larger number of references was deemed appropriate. In Chapter 9 we draw together the common themes across the various clinical and management areas covered in the previous chapters. We also attempt to look into the near future and anticipate the ethical issues that will be raised by new developments in speech and language therapy provision.

A list of the areas not covered in the book might turn out to be longer than the book itself, but we should note some of the absences made unavoidable by limitations of space. In terms of client groups, we were unable to include scenarios specifically based on dysfluency, voice, cleft palate, neonatal feeding or mental health, to name but a few, and we recognise that all these areas of clinical practice have the potential to present significant ethical challenges. Our hope is that the issues that are discussed in relation to our scenarios translate to other client groups. We also decided not to include the ethics of research in relation to speech and language therapy. Although there have been steady increases over the last few years in both the importance attached to research and the number of clinicians involved in it, the profile of clinical ethics seemed to us to be in greater need of development at present. This reflects a sentiment expressed, by way of example, in the UK Royal College of Speech and Language Therapists' (RCSLT) *Communicating Quality 3*: 'With the advent of clinical governance, health professionals are being increasingly called upon to examine the ethics that lie behind all practice decisions' (RCSLT, 2006, p. 15).

Finally, we inevitably need to acknowledge that not everyone will agree with everything written in the book. Although we have not set out to provide prescriptive solutions to the situations described in the scenarios, various viewpoints and courses of action are offered by the commentators and by us. That these may not meet with universal agreement reflects the essence of the subject matter of the book. As Malec (1993) says in a discussion of ethical approaches to (brain injury) rehabilitation, 'a fundamentally shared value in a pluralistic society is that many values need not be shared' (p. 384). Beauchamp and Childress (2009) put this even more strongly, saying, 'we regard disunity, conflict, and moral ambiguity as pervasive features of the moral life' (p. 374). Despite this acknowledgement, it is important that discussion of ethical issues should not serve to make situations even less comprehensible than before the discussion. To quote Peter Carey in his novel *Theft: A Love Story* (2006), 'There is so much fog around the moral high ground' (p. 155). We hope that our discussions render the fog somewhat less impenetrable.

2 Practising ethically

Introduction

In this chapter we review a number of key concepts in healthcare ethics in order to inform the discussion of clinical scenarios later in the book. We also consider other resources and strategies that may, in theory at least, be used to assist SLTs to reflect on and deal with ethical issues in practice. In terms of concepts, we discuss the current dominant medical ethics approach, first described by Beauchamp and Childress 30 years ago and now published in a sixth edition (2009), consider some of the criticisms levelled at this type of approach, and introduce alternative approaches. Beauchamp and Childress's principles have attracted much discussion and broad-based acceptance in medical circles, to the extent that they are now often referred to simply as 'the four principles'. Not everyone agrees, however, that principlism offers the most useful conceptual approach. We review a range of alternatives, including the ethics of care, virtue ethics and Seedhouse's Foundations Theory of Health, together with associated concepts that are important for understanding the field as a whole. In terms of other resources, we examine the content, structure and function of codes of ethics, together with their strengths, benefits and limitations, and then deal with decision-making protocols, often devised with a view to helping health professionals apply ethical thinking to real situations. Finally we consider what it might mean to think and act ethically in a proactive manner, as a routine part of daily practice.

Before launching ourselves into theories of bioethics, we should first mention the wider sphere of moral philosophy that serves as much of the source material for those theories. More precisely, we should explain why we do not provide coverage of this in the book. What we are (not) talking about here is the work of moral philosophers such as Kant, Hobbes, Mill and Sartre, together with concepts like utilitariansim, existentialism and deontology. That body of work is both important and influential (though the list above represents a distinctly Eurocentric perspective) but is less immediately applicable to the field of therapy we are interested in than the approaches to healthcare ethics specifically which we describe below. As Sokol (2006) puts it, 'An encyclopaedic knowledge of the works of the great moral philosophers will not necessarily translate into a helpful and insightful case analysis' (p. 1226). In fact, Cowley (2005) goes further than that, asserting that the use of terms such as 'consequentialism', 'deontology' and even 'the four principles' as the jargon of medical ethics 'can lead student and practitioner into ignoring their own healthy ethical intuitions and vocabulary' (p. 739). Moral philosophy is also a body of work well described by other people (see, e.g., Wilmot, 1997), both in its 'pure' form and in its reinterpretation in relation to medical ethics.

Principles and other conceptual approaches to ethics

'Ethics needs principles – four can encompass the rest', declares the title of an article by medical ethicist Raanan Gillon (2003). In the opposite corner, however, we have a distinctly different take: 'The four principles approach is manifestly empty, and has achieved its great popularity as a direct result' (Seedhouse, 1998, p. 130). At least Beauchamp and Childress can be assured that their work has not faded into obscurity. The existence of such strongly opposing views is itself evidence of the degree to which the principles are entrenched in bioethical thinking. Before we discuss the origins of the principles and how they have been used in healthcare in general, we should explain briefly what they are taken to mean.

Autonomy

Seen by Gillon (2003) as the 'first among equals' of the four ethics principles (p. 307), and by McLean and Mason (2003) as having become 'the trumping ethical value in the last 50 years or so' (p. 47), autonomy is described by Beauchamp and Childress (2009), who incidentally do not themselves assert its priority, as 'self-rule that is free from controlling interference by others and from certain limitations such as an inadequate understanding that prevents meaningful choice' (p. 99). The principle of autonomy is therefore primarily interpreted as support for people being free (and able) to decide for themselves. It is commonly associated with consent to treatment, and lends itself to discussion of what constitutes informed consent. The notion of freedom from controlling interference referred to by Beauchamp and Childress could refer to interference from any number of players – family, friends, health workers, bank managers, politicians – all of whom can take actions that serve to restrict a specific decision; limitations that prevent meaningful choice would encompass social influences (e.g. socioeconomic status) and more directly physical influences, examples being states of restricted consciousness such as coma, of restricted cognition such as dementia, or of restricted communication such as difficulty with comprehension.

   Seedhouse (1998) makes a strong case for autonomy to be seen as much more than the right of people to make their own choices. He distinguishes, on the one hand, the obligation for health workers to work towards creating and enhancing patients' autonomy and, on the other, the obligation to respect their choices, the point between these being said to represent an 'autonomy flip' (i.e. a tipping point between the two). This goes much further than the notion that informed choice is just about giving people enough information to *make* a choice. One of Seedhouse's examples illustrates this point more easily. If health workers override a depressed patient's resistance to social activity by continuing to provide social opportunities, they might be ignoring the patient's immediate autonomous wish on a relatively superficial level but may still be working justifiably towards a deeper kind of autonomy, since the patient may ultimately be more fulfilled by working his or her way out of the depression.

Nonmaleficence

The principle of nonmaleficence refers to the obligation not to harm people or to subject them to the risk of harm (by negligence) and is paraphrased neatly by Colicutt McGrath (2007) as 'Don't make things worse' (p. 85). It is generally seen as a stronger obligation than beneficence (described below), in that we are under greater moral expectation not to harm people than we are to actively help them. Having said that, it is also seen as being (in general) easier to accomplish by virtue of requiring us simply to refrain from action. The interpretation of the seemingly straightforward injunction not to harm people depends itself on interpretation of what constitutes harm in particular circumstances, and this in turn depends on what values people hold. It also comes into potential conflict with the principle of beneficence, where, for example, it is deemed necessary to administer short-term harm (e.g. surgery) for predicted longer-term gain. Similarly, removing a service from one group of people in order to shift resources to another (possibly larger) group of people involves what might be seen as a necessary harm. In medicine the principle of nonmaleficence comes to the fore in debates about abortion and assisted dying. In speech and language therapy it might apply, say, to provision of a language disorder screening programme where there is no facility for providing intervention after identification.

Beneficence

The principle of beneficence refers to the obligation to do good and to balance potential risks and benefits in favour of a person's welfare. It seems reasonable to assume that notions of beneficence are central to people's thought processes when they decide to take up a career in speech and language therapy and other health professions. As noted above, the obligations of beneficence are felt to be less strong than those of nonmaleficence, not least because there are an infinite number of good deeds that we could do for other people whereas nonmaleficence requires us to do as few bad deeds as possible. However, similar difficulties arise with the interpretation of beneficence as with nonmaleficence: what I think is good for you may not equate to what you think is good for you. This conflict is expressed in medical ethics literature in terms of paternalism, i.e. where a patient's autonomy is in conflict with what the health professional deems the most beneficent action.

The field of psychiatry, for example, is particularly ripe for this kind of conflict, especially where involuntary hospitalisation is concerned. One important aspect of the general principle of beneficence is that obligations are seen to become greater where there is some sort of special relationship. In other words, we are expected to put ourselves out more for family, friends and, most importantly for our purposes, patients than we are for people with no special claim on our lives.

Justice

Distributive justice (as opposed to corrective or punitive justice, with which we are not concerned here) is defined as 'fair, equitable, and appropriate distribution' (Beauchamp & Childress, 2009, p. 241) and is the principle that underlies allocation of healthcare resources. Problems of resource allocation, and therefore of justice, are said to arise in conditions of scarcity and competition, and it is not difficult to see how the prevalence of these circumstances underscores the importance of this principle in healthcare decision making. As with the other principles, there seems to be something innately important about this kind of justice, in that we all wish be treated at least equally with other people, but problems again arise when more exact definition is attempted. For example, the actual needs of a six-year-old child with a stutter are very difficult to compare with those of a woman in her forties with Huntington's chorea: it therefore makes little sense to assert that they should receive exactly the same resources. A large amount of work has gone into developing workable interpretations of this basic principle (e.g. QALYs – Quality Adjusted Life Years – and the work of John Rawls [1971] and its subsequent application specifically to health by Norman Daniels [1985]), and we return to these ideas at various points in the book (in particular Chapter 8).

In addition to these four superordinate principles, Beauchamp and Childress (2009) list a number of related concepts. Although these are not put forward by the authors themselves as principles, they are sometimes reinterpreted by others as such (see, e,g., the discussion of codes of ethics below). These concepts include veracity (telling the truth), fidelity (acting in good faith) and confidentiality. As with the four principles, the concepts pose challenges of interpretation. For example, although telling the truth may be a behaviour generally expected of healthcare professionals by the public, it might not necessarily be a good idea to tell the (whole) truth to someone who may in some way be harmed by the news (thereby violating the principle of nonmaleficence). (We look in detail at the issue of defining and imparting truth in Chapter 7.) Fidelity refers to actions such as keeping promises and fulfilling responsibilities, and is of relevance to conflicts of interest (say between a child's perceived needs and the parents' wishes). Finally, confiden-tiality – a term in widespread use and thus very familiar to health professionals – does not, for instance, sit easily with another familiar concept, teamworking.

According to Beauchamp and Childress, the principles provide general and comprehensive moral norms which serve as a starting point for the delineation of more specific rules. The fact that the principles can conflict with each other, for instance when doing good by overriding someone's autonomy, is seen as a positive and realistic reflection of the complexity of moral life. The inevitable consequence is that the principles (together with associated rules, rights, virtues and ideals) 'do not function as precise guides to action that direct us in each circumstance' (Beauchamp & Childress, 2009, p. 13) (though Beauchamp and Childress complete this sentence with the phrase 'in the way that more detailed rules and judgments do'). Unfortunately, what is one person's (or set of authors') proviso or caution is red rag to another. Seedhouse (1998) follows his earlier statement on the manifest emptiness of the four principles approach with a further dismissal: 'Because the principles lack detail – and since their adherents' attempted justifications swiftly collapse into waffle – they can be used by almost anyone to defend almost anything' (p. 130). Similarly, Harris (2003) suggests that the four principles constitute little more than a checklist of things to consider (which, he acknowledges, might be useful for those who are new to the field of bioethics). Moreover, he asserts that if everyone subscribed to the principles as a means to address ethical decisions, it would lead to 'sterility and uniformity of approach of a quite mindbogglingly boring kind' (p. 303) – though it is not clear from this why boredom is a relevant or necessarily negative attribute of any system.

So, there are some fundamental differences of opinion on the part of medical ethicists as to the value of identifying four principles and the uses to which they can be put. Further discussion of these opposing positions is not within the scope of this book but we do need to recognise that, despite significant criticism, the four principles (and related concepts from the work of Beauchamp and Childress) have permeated all areas of Western medical ethics thinking and have been used as the foundation for many professional codes of ethics, including those within speech and language therapy. We now turn to the rather different perspective offered by a conceptual approach called the ethics of care. Although this has not arisen from healthcare, or been applied systematically to it, the ethics of care is concerned with issues of relationship that make it worthy of reflection with regard to the nature of speech and language therapy work.

The ethics of care

The ethics of care (also termed care ethics) as a specific approach has its origins in work by feminist theorists, including Carol Gilligan (1982), Joan Tronto (1993) and Nel Noddings (2003). It arose partly in response to the fact that care and caring relationships, despite their importance in our lives, have largely been ignored by moral philosophers, and partly as an alternative to what were seen as primarily male ways of interpreting the world.

Tronto (1993) identifies four phases of care and, arising from these, four ethical elements of care. The phases she posits are 'caring about', which involves recognising that care is required; 'taking care of', in which someone assumes responsibility for the need that has been recognised; 'care-giving', in which the care needs are addressed (either successfully or not); and 'care-receiving', which focuses on the response of the recipient of care. The four associated ethical elements of care are attentiveness, responsibility, competence and responsiveness. Attentiveness to the potential needs of others is a prerequisite for meeting those needs. Responsibility is described by Tronto as a central moral category where people make a choice whether to attend to an identified care need or not. Here the notion of choice calls to mind Seedhouse's (1998) use of the term 'deliberation' with regard to how to act in relation to other people (see Chapter 1). We, as private individuals and as SLTs, are constantly faced with choices of action in relation to other people's (care) needs, which have ethical implications. The third ethical element, competence, refers to the fact that it is not enough to recognise a care need and accept responsibility for it if that need is ultimately not met. Competence therefore provides for a focus on the outcome of care, to be assessed as far as possible in terms of the responses of the recipient of care – or 'cared-for' in Noddings' terminology. This is represented by the final element, responsiveness, which turns the focus of attention onto the cared-for and 'enables the practitioner to understand the person's experience, providing the opportunity, when necessary, to change care to make it more suitable' (Brannelly, 2006, p. 201). 'Encourages' might be a more realistic word than 'enables' here, given the challenge of interpreting the experiences of people with severe cognitive or communication impairment.

Cockburn (2005) summarises the main differences between the ethics of care and what is sometimes called the 'ethics of rights', i.e. the approach taken by exponents of Beauchamp and Childress's work. As well as emphasising responsibilities and relationships rather than rules and rights, the ethics of care is said to be linked to concrete situations (rather than being abstract), focuses on people's feelings and opinions, and is conceptualised as a moral activity rather than a set of principles. An approach based on rights is seen as fundamentally adversarial, in that ethical dilemmas become a context to find the predominant principle, whereas 'the moral repertoire also needs to include principles of cooperation, intimacy, trust, connection and compassion to be emphasized as important sources of moral reasoning' (Cockburn, 2005, p. 78). Another way of looking at this is that while the principles approach to medical ethics emphasises individualism and autonomy via the actions and obligations of individual moral agents, the ethics of care takes a rather different stance by focusing on the care relationship itself, including the roles of the people caring and those who are cared for. To paraphrase Slote (2007), the principles approach emphasises autonomy *from* other individuals (and the just application of principles to support it) whereas the ethics of care focuses on connection *to* others. Although it comes from a completely different field, Clark's (1996) work on conversation as a form of joint action might help to illustrate this. Clark describes conversation as one subtype of the many and varied joint actions that people perform – he gives examples such as rowing a boat with someone else and playing a duet – that cannot be understood without recognising the roles of all the participants as well as the dynamic and interdependent relationship between them. The ethics of care is concerned with a special type of joint activity but is similarly founded on recognition of the roles of all the participants in care relationships and on the nature of the relationship itself, as well as foregrounding the centrality of care to human lives.

As noted above, the ethics of care originated in the field of (feminist) politics and it has continued to be discussed in relation to the political world. It has also been applied extensively to the field of education, particularly through the work of Noddings (1988, 2003), and to a lesser extent to social care. Discussion of the ethics of care within health has been slower to develop. One example of a field of medicine where the potential of the ethics of care has been noted is psychiatry. Adshead (2002) notes that the ethics of care is particularly relevant in psychiatry because 'therapeutic relationships are themselves the vehicle of treatment' (p. 56), a view that resonates with much of speech and language therapy practice. She writes further that 'ethical debates . . . which focus solely on conflicts between two principles . . . cannot address the complexity of the lives of individuals, and the relationships in which they are embedded' (p. 56). This perspective on psychiatry, that it is an uncomfortable fit with the most widely promoted approach to medical ethics, may shed some light on a description of the discipline as a bioethical ugly duckling (Fulford & Hope, 1993) and may also illustrate why bioethical principles and speech and language therapy may not be an entirely comfortable fit either. Adshead (2002) argues that in fact there are situations in the whole of medicine where the therapeutic relationship is the vehicle of treatment and that this is where the ethics of care is more relevant than bioethical principles.

As is the case for the principles approach, the status and appropriateness of the ethics of care in relation to health are subject to disagreement. Allmark (2002) argues strongly that the concept of care is too vague and underspecified to be practically useful, backing up his argument via discussion of the overlapping and confusing meanings of derived terms such as 'careful', 'careless' and 'uncaring'. He takes issue with the central status accorded the parent–child (in most writing, mother–child) relationship in the development of ethics of care theory. Although it may seem intuitively attractive that (good) caring between parents and children provides some sort of template for morally good relationships between people in general, Allmark argues that there is no clear reason why other aspects of parent–child relationships, such as hate or jealousy, could not equally serve as a template. His conclusion is represented by the argument that '*what* [our italics] we care about is morally important, the fact that we care *per se* is not' (p. 68). It is also important to note that it is not clear how ethics of care might be operationalised in relation to any particular ethical issue.

We have highlighted the ethics of care here primarily as a possible counterbalance to the predominance of thinking based on the principles approach, particularly because of its grounding in narratives of complex interactions and connections. We suggest that it may be something to keep in mind during the remainder of the book.

Virtue ethics

Another approach that emphasises the importance of giving weight to emotion in our ethical deliberations is found in virtue ethics. Gardiner (2003) suggests that 'emotions are not to be accepted as instinctive unmanageable reactions but as sensitivities that inform our judgments' (p. 298). For the virtue ethicist, what is important is the character of, say, the therapist contemplating a difficult ethical decision, rather than any disembodied (and potentially conflicting) principles relating to actions.

In fact, the interpretations of virtue ethics found in healthcare literature attempt to move the focus of ethical thinking away from ethical dilemmas and decision making on the basis that 'it is both a practical and logical error to examine break-down situations and assume that the analysis depicts the same processes that occur in excellent practice' (Brenner, 1997, p. 51). A variety of possible virtues can be identified. Beauchamp and Childress themselves identify five virtues, namely trustworthiness, integrity, discernment, compassion and conscientiousness. Gardiner discusses the original virtues put forward by ancient Greek philosophers: courage, prudence, temperance and justice, and also considers some theologically based virtues – faith, hope and charity. The variety of candidates for consideration again suggests that while the theory and concepts might be relevant to health-care discussions, converting them directly into clinical practice might not be a straightforward process.

The Foundations Theory of Health

The Foundations Theory of Health, described by Seedhouse and co-authors in various publications (Seedhouse, 1998, 2001, 2002b; Wright-St Clair & Seedhouse, 2005), is not a theory of ethics as such but a theory of the purpose of healthcare, which according to its author provides the foundation for morally good healthcare work. Although the theory has not been subjected to extensive debate in medical ethics circles (and certainly not to the extent that the principles approach has), it represents a different perspective on how to arrive at ethically sound practice. By starting with the fundamental question '*Why* do we work for people's health?', the theory can prompt thinking and debate about a variety of related ethical questions.

Seedhouse (2002) describes work for health thus:

> *It is a question of providing the appropriate foundations to enable the achievement of personal and group potentials. Health . . . is created by removing obstacles and by providing the basic means by which biological and chosen goals can be achieved. (p. 94)*

He lists the most important foundations required for a person's health as basic needs (e.g. food, shelter), access to information about factors that influence that person's life, skill and confidence to understand and manipulate the information, and finally recognition that individuals (and therefore their potentials and goals) are never completely isolated from other people. The fourth foundation, which is based around belonging and community, is said to involve such things as awareness of one's dependence on other people and of the duty to support others. In fact, even the first foundation containing basic needs is not restricted to physical needs but also includes purpose in life (Wright-St Clair & Seedhouse, 2005). Seedhouse employs the image of these four areas as building blocks (and extends the analogy into the requirements for good building work), with a fifth building block being required at some times by some people. It is the fifth block that contains (among other things) health services as we know them, the services set up to meet what we routinely think of as health needs. What is particularly important in this conception is that it establishes the four building blocks, including moral awareness, as (absolute) requirements for health, supplemented as required by what we term 'health' services. A final point worth noting (and which is relevant to the issues discussed in Chapter 6) is that Seedhouse makes no distinction between tangible obstacles (such as unavailability of medicines) and mental obstacles (such as a family's lack of understanding of the situation confronting them) but classifies them all as limitations to potential and thus as barriers to health.

Before we move on to look at the content and function of speech and language therapy codes of ethics, it is worth highlighting a number of other concepts which are the subject of topical debate in healthcare ethics and are thus of relevance in consideration of ethics in speech and language therapy.

Bioethics and healthcare ethics

We use the term *healthcare ethics* in this book (in preference to medical ethics or bioethics) for two reasons. The first is that it is a more inclusive term that is relevant to speech and language therapy as well as medicine (and a better proposition than 'allied health ethics' or 'speech and language therapy ethics'). In other words, with it we can encompass all aspects of ethics applied to healthcare (including the areas that come under medical ethics and bioethics). The second, related reason is that healthcare ethics does not imply a medical model for approaching ethical issues. This is in line with the view of Fulford et al. (2002), who draw a distinction between the terms healthcare ethics and bioethics which highlights fundamentally different approaches. For them, bioethics is representative of the medical model found in secondary care services (e.g. hospitals), characterised by a focus on a specific subset of values, on fact-based and reasoning-based approaches to the provision of health services, and by an emphasis on ethics as a tool for regulation (see below). Healthcare ethics, they propose, is an approach that is concerned with more than just regulation, an approach that incorporates values as well as facts and that recognises the importance of a diversity of values. In fact, the recognition of such diversity of values serves to place the need for good communication at the heart of Fulford et al.'s conceptualisation, in order that people can understand what each other's values are.

Regulatory ethics

The origins of bioethics as a response to rapid developments in medicine and to misuses of medical power gave it a natural regulatory, quasi-legal function. 'Biotechnology, in itself morally neutral, was seen as being in need of control if it was to be directed to good purposes rather than bad' (Fulford et al., 2002, p. 2). Although regulation may have been, and may to some extent remain, a natural function of ethical debate, there have been reactions against this as the sole purpose of ethics. Recognition of the need for ethical thinking in healthcare to take into account a diversity of values is not necessarily compatible with a central tendency towards regulation (something we return to in the discussion of codes of ethics below). In addition, over-regulation (seen most clearly in the sometimes labyrinthine processes of research ethics review) is seen as being at odds with healthcare in the real world. This is particularly the case where healthcare is undertaken in the community and is difficult to regulate. Finally, the power of service users continues to rise as people gain more access to health knowledge, and as the assumption decreases that health professionals inherently know best and should therefore function as regulators.

Power

Health professionals, including SLTs, are in an inherently powerful position in relation to people using health services, by virtue of differentials in knowledge and skills, health need and status, among others. Although the same might be said to apply to anyone who has or does something that someone else needs, the centrality of health to our lives accentuates this relationship. Over and above these basic aspects of power imbalance are additional complicating factors such as age (health interactions with children and older people), culture (where a patient's cultural affiliations are not adequately represented in the healthcare workforce or cultural practices are not respected) and of course the challenges posed by sensory, motor, cognitive and communication impairment. Despite this inherent disequilibrium, the concept of power does not feature frequently in discussions of healthcare ethics in general and ethical principles in particular.

  Brody (2002) suggests that the sharing of power between people providing health services and those using them 'constitutes an important ethical safeguard within the relationship' and that 'there are some special benefits to be gained from . . . putting the term *power* back into the vocabulary of medical ethics' (p. 133). This sentiment is reflected in moves to empower, say, people with aphasia (see Chapter 5) and could reasonably be predicted to increase not only patients' sense of control but also their engagement with therapy and their compliance – a word unfortunately replete with connotations of power – with therapy decisions, since these would be the result of informed negotiation anyway. Although the importance accorded to patient autonomy within the principles approach might appear to have the potential to address the power imbalance, Brody argues that a better way to address this imbalance is via the construction of joint narratives by clinician and patient that allow the patient to develop a new life story as required.

Objectivism and relativism

Finally in this section we take a brief look at the two opposing concepts of objectivism and relativism. Although this takes us into the realms of 'pure' moral theory outside the world of healthcare (where we claimed in the introduction to the chapter we would not be going), the relationship between these two concepts is of importance for health professionals, particularly in cross-cultural interactions, and is relevant to the discussion of codes of ethics that follows.

From the perspective of objectivism, there are fundamental truths – notions of right and wrong – which proponents assert should apply to everyone. Views at this end of the continuum might conceivably be based in religious belief or respect for longstanding tradition (Macklin, 1999). The relativist viewpoint, on the other end, suggests that since views vary across cultures, societies and individuals, there can be no fundamental truths about what is right or wrong and thus ethics is entirely dependent on time and place. The upshot of this is that all views become intrinsically worthy of tolerance and respect and nothing can legitimately be declared 'wrong'. One frequent argument levelled against the relativist view in its strongest form is that even acts such as genocide cannot logically be condemned. However, Macklin (1999) proposes that a case can be made for a modified form of ethical relativism on the basis that 'some ethical matters deal with basic ways human beings treat each other, whereas others shade into what is more like etiquette' (p. 11). On this basis, whereas the infliction of bodily harm or restriction of freedom might be seen as universally closer to being ethically 'wrong', different cultural attitudes to, say, personal privacy might be closer to culturally based etiquette.

The reason that the continuum between objectivism and relativism is important in relation to healthcare is that, in their professional lives at least, people working in healthcare in societies with any degree of multiculturalism cannot reasonably take either extreme ethical position. If the provision of healthcare is based on monolithic objectivist 'truths', then people who do not share those views will be wary of taking up the service (and since the aim of health services is presumably to facilitate better health for everyone, this would be self-defeating). Rowson (2006) outlines three reasons that healthcare cannot be based on extreme relativist views either. Firstly, professions need to agree on at least *some* basic shared values to avoid widely varying individual responses to the same health issue. Secondly, professions need to state shared values that are deemed worthwhile by the community. That way, potential recipients of the service, whatever their cultural background, know what to expect and, it is hoped, can trust practitioners to adhere to the stated values. Finally, a profession needs the goodwill of the society in which it works, and it will only achieve this 'if its members strive to comply with values that are generally thought to be in the interests of society as a whole' (Rowson, 2006, p. 42). Public inquiry tends to be the end result when that goodwill goes seriously astray.

The notion of a statement of shared values has as its main outlet professional codes of ethics, which we discuss in the next section.

Codes of ethics

Speech and language therapy institutional codes of ethics generally take as their starting point the principles described by Beauchamp and Childress over the last 30 years, and then either modify or expand them. For example, the Speech

Pathology Australia (SPA) (2000) code lists the four principles described above and adds truth and professional integrity to the list. These are described as the basis for decision making. The Code of Ethics of the UK Royal College of Speech and Language Therapists (RCSLT) (2006) presents a broadly similar picture. It is described as being grounded in '*the* [our italics] broad ethical principles of healthcare', which is of note in itself for the implication that these principles are so well established as to warrant the definite article. The principles in the RCSLT code are supplemented by what are termed values of personal and professional integrity, a commitment to competent and effective practice, care for the individual, inclusion and teamworking.

The standard approach of supplementing Beauchamp and Childress's principles is thus to provide further ethical concepts labelled either as principles themselves or as values. Despite commonalities, the full codes of the various institutional bodies differ in emphasis and tone, particularly in relation to their use of aspirational language. The Preamble to the Code of Ethics of the American Speech-Language-Hearing Association (ASHA) (2003) refers to the underlying principles as 'aspirational and inspirational in nature' (p. 1), though the rules in the code tend towards proscriptive phrasing. For example, Principle I, Rule L states, 'Individuals shall not reveal, without authorization, any professional or personal information about identified persons served professionally' (p. 2), and then specifies exclusions based on the welfare of the client or community and legal requirements.

SPA (2000) takes a more overtly aspirational stance by encouraging members to consider what is ethical in fulfilling a range of duties and to aspire to ethical conduct, rather than simply avoiding unethical behaviour. For example, in the section on professional competence the SPA code – written collectively in the first person – states that 'we . . . strive continually to update and extend our professional knowledge and skills through such activities as attending professional development, seeking a mentor or seeking supervision' (p. 4). However, even here it is not possible to avoid proscription altogether:

> We do not disclose information about our clients, or the confidences they share with us, unless: our clients consent to this; the law requires us to disclose it; or there are compelling moral and ethical reasons for us to disclose it. (p. 4)

Taking a step to one side for a moment, it is worth considering how Alison in Chapter 1 might interpret the statements from ASHA and SPA on disclosure of information in the light of her confidentiality dilemma.

Given that the various national bodies representing speech and language therapists each have one, the obvious question is 'What are codes of ethics for?' Here we highlight two functions which codes might fulfil: a public statement of a profession's values (and/or standards) and a measure against which standards of individual performance (particularly transgressions) can be judged. After consideration of these functions, we discuss some of the possible limitations and disadvantages of codes of ethics.

Chabon and Ulrich (2006), in a discussion on the ASHA website, describe a code of ethics as

a shared statement of the values specific to a particular group. It defines, and makes public, common fundamental principles and standards for practice, research, and education; supports self-reflection and public accountability; and recognizes individuals as a community of professionals with unique privileges and obligations.

This idea of a statement of values is reflected in the codes of various professional associations, including those of: Canada – 'the fundamental values and standards essential to . . . responsible practice' (Canadian Association of Speech-Language Pathologists and Audiologists, 2005, p. 1); South Africa – 'the highest possible standards of practice' (South African Speech-Language-Hearing Association, 1997, p. 1); and New Zealand – 'the highest standards of integrity and ethical principles' (New Zealand Speech-Language Therapists' Association, 2000, p. 3) – as well as those outlined above. Chabon and Ulrich (2006) suggest that codes present a context for decision making that is different from the perspectives of public opinion and the law or the views of individuals. As we discuss below, there is limited support for the idea that codes of ethics can facilitate detailed decision making but more widespread support for the idea that, by making a statement of values and standards, they can act as a *context* which promotes good ethical conduct.

The promotion of a good ethical context is intended to affect (or indeed improve) the behaviour of professionals and thus to have potential benefits for the public as recipients of speech and language therapy services. According to Parsons (2004), writing about the profession of public relations, a code of ethics can act as a 'profession's contract with the society it serves' (p. 68) by setting out the values and standards that guide members' services to and interactions with members of the public. Fisher (2003), writing in similar vein about the aims of psychologists' codes of ethics, describes a code as 'a contract with society to act in consumers' best interests' (p. 7) and as a set of standards against which professionals can be held accountable. Codes can therefore provide good public relations for professions (Wright-St Clair & Seedhouse, 2005), one aspect of the way a profession presents itself. Although one view of public relations is that it might benefit the profession rather than the patients, a more positive interpretation would be that professions recognise the importance of (a) having an ethical standpoint and (b) providing those outside the profession with the opportunity to assess both the standpoint and the profession's (and individual practitioners') adherence to it. This, of course, assumes that the codes of ethics are easily accessible by the public.

This takes us to the second potential function, that of providing 'rules that articulate *enforceable* [our italics] standards, expectations and proscriptions' (Chabon & Ulrich, 2006). Sim (1997) notes that the professional body has the responsibility for writing the code and then promulgating and enforcing it. SPA states that its code of ethics provides standards by which people can evaluate the profession from the outside. Codes of ethics are the usual starting point for members of the public who wish to make a complaint about a professional. The words 'conduct' and 'behaviour' (and in some cases 'violation') tend to crop up in the various codes.

Although, as Fisher (2003) discusses, codes can have some role in the enforcement of ethical behaviour through clear delineation of types of behaviour that consitute ethical violations, the fact that codes are brought into play when professionals are disciplined for their behaviour suggests that the enforcement is generally retrospective (i.e. the violation has occurred). Not surprisingly, none of the associations claims that its code is anything other than a starting point in any disciplinary process, and some, such as SPA, do not use the code of ethics to refer to this at all.

The other side of the code of ethics coin features a number of limitations and possible disadvantages. For a start, any potential capacity that codes might have to guide ethical practice is predicated on the assumption that the standards and values articulated in them are collectively agreed and represent a consensus of values, what Fisher (2003) calls a 'community of common purpose' (p. 6). This is not necessarily the case, and in situations where members' standards and interpretations differ from some assumed professional, cultural norm, ethics boards tend to be charged with responsibility for resolving the differences.

If, as noted above, codes of ethics are seen as too blunt a tool to support detailed disciplinary proceedings, they are also acknowledged to be of limited use for clinicians faced with specific ethical challenges. According to the Canadian Association of Speech-Language Pathologists and Audiologists (2005), its code 'cannot offer definitive resolution to all ethical questions that may arise during professional practice' (p. 1).

There are several reasons for this state of affairs. Most obviously, codes of ethics have to be written in general terms, at odds with the specifics of clinical situations. If we think back to the situation in which Alison finds herself at the beginning of Chapter 1, wondering whether to divulge sensitive information to colleagues without explicit permission, we can see that she is unlikely to be helped in her decision by referring to a code of ethics. Although she will doubtless want to take beneficent action in order to 'do good' for the child, it is not at all clear which action will do the most good. Similarly, an argument could be made for several courses of action as the most effective way to avoid harm to either the child or her mother (or indeed the father, about whom relatively little is known for certain). Finally, recognition of the importance of autonomy would probably support at least discussing possible disclosure with the mother and possibly handing her the decision in full, but this may not result in the 'best' outcome for the child. As we have already noted, statements about confidentiality are also likely to be too general to help Alison come to a decision.

Rules which attempt to set down what should and should not be done in all circumstances quickly become outdated. Further, mandated ethics do not assist clinicians to recognise or understand the complex and relational nature of ethical issues in their work; what is 'ethical' is embedded in the nature of the relationship between client and clinician. Biomedically derived codes place limited emphasis on the relational nature of practice, given that biomedical work may entail little or limited interaction between patient and clinician. Codes of ethics in allied health professions, derived as they are from a biomedical model of practice, risk overlooking this key factor.

At this point it is worth returning to consider the ethics of care. As we have discussed, it emphasises not the individual rights- or duty-based actions of isolated, individual moral agents (for our purposes, SLTs) but the relationships of care between people. As Noddings (1988) says, the primary concern of moral agents is 'the relation itself – not only what happens physically to others involved in the relation and in connected relations but what they may feel and how they may respond to the act under consideration' (p. 219). It may be particularly relevant that 'traditional moral philosophy has overlooked the contributions of the cared-for' – in our case the patients and carers interacting with SLTs – 'because these contributions cannot always be described in terms of moral agency or adherence to principle' (Noddings, 2003, p. xiv). In this approach what is deemed important is the ethical quality of the relationship of care rather than the good or bad actions of either party. It is not difficult to see that biomedically driven codes of ethics might struggle to represent such a different perspective. According to Brannelly (2006), when practitioners accept responsibility for someone, their work 'moves beyond the stated minimum standards required by, for example, professional bodies, to a personal, and perhaps emotional involvement that is necessary to care well' (p. 200).

Wright-St Clair and Seedhouse (2005) argue that attempts to codify professional behaviour and biomedical ethics have flourished in environments of technological developments, consumer sophistication and increased public scrutiny of health professionals, which have led to public and professional 'fascination in extraordinary events' (p. 19) when something happens to bring the commonplace invisible nature of morality into sharp relief. They highlight the danger of having codes that stand as a public statement of a profession's philosophy and values without impacting on moral behaviour. To use their assertion, 'ethical codes are predominantly mute on the matter of moral competence' (p. 20). Beauchamp and Childress (2009) also recognise this danger, stating that 'professionals may mistakenly suppose that they satisfy all relevant moral requirements if they obediently follow the rules of the code' (p. 7).

Even if we accept – as we certainly do – that ethics is intrinsic to all healthcare work, there will still be circumstances in which the issues take the form of a 'classical' dilemma. If codes of ethics do not provide detailed practical guidance on how to act ethically in a specific situation, are there other tools that can perform this function?

Ethical decision-making protocols

There is no shortage of tools that purport to facilitate the process of ethical decision making. Some have been developed from a broad perspective on healthcare in general, others from specific clinical areas such as brain injury or specific professions such as nursing or indeed speech and language therapy. The overview that follows is intended only to be sufficient to allow some general conclusions to be drawn.

A parsimonious description of ethical decision-making protocols in general would be that they attempt to break down the process of considering an ethical issue into sequential steps along the lines of 'What are the key issues?', 'What are the possible courses of action?' and 'What would be the consequences of each action?' An exception to this approach is Seedhouse's (1998) ethical grid, which we discuss later. First we give a brief description of some of the step-by-step models from speech and language therapy and elsewhere.

One illustration of the step-by-step approach is the DECIDE model proposed by Thompson, Melia and Boyd (2000) in their book on ethics in nursing. The acronym DECIDE prompts users to define the problem, ethically review, consider the options, investigate outcomes, decide on action and evaluate the results of that action. The authors further subcategorise these six steps in the ethical decision-making process into three consecutive pairs representing (a) consideration of the background *causes*, (b) appraisal of the potential *means* for addressing the issue and (c) action towards appropriate *ends*.

Similar factors are covered by Colicutt McGrath (2007) for people working in the field of brain injury in what she terms a heuristic for managing ethical dilemmas. This provides a flow diagram with labels such as 'List all interested parties', 'Locate points of conflict' and 'Brainstorm relevant courses of action' (p. 114). Both this and the previous model emphasise that although they are essentially sequential in nature, they should be used iteratively with recursion to previous stages as required.

Attempts to produce practical ways of working through ethical issues are in constant development, as our third model illustrates. Sokol (2008) presents for (re)consideration the 'four quadrants' approach to clinical ethics case analysis, an approach first put forward by Jonsen, Siegler and Winslade (1982) (now in a sixth edition) and used widely in America but less in some other countries. The four quadrants prompt the user to address particular areas in sequence, the first being the medical indications in the case under consideration (though for our non-medical purposes this section could just as easily be thought of as clinical indications). This would cover diagnosis, likely outcome of any interventions, etc. The second quadrant takes in the patient's expressed preferences towards courses of action; the third quadrant prompts the user to consider the effect on quality of life of courses of action, and the final quadrant highlights contextual features.

Sokol (2008) contrasts the four quadrants approach with the four principles by suggesting that whereas the latter operate at 'mid-level' across a whole situation, the four quadrants 'operate very close to the action, asking questions of immediate relevance to the case at hand' (p. 516). They also encourage clinicians, once they have immersed themselves 'elbow deep' in the key medical/clinical facts, to gradually zoom out to take in the wider perspectives of the patient's life. This approach is certainly based on a logical progression of thinking that should come readily to most clinicians. The prompts, on the other hand, are only very broadly specified and the model is designed for (medical) ethical dilemmas where there may be relatively clear competing courses of action.

It is fair to say that these models provide a logical sequence to problem solving which can be a useful starting point and can provide a sense of control, particularly for inexperienced clinicians, in what can otherwise feel like an amorphous mass of issues and possibilities. Protocols also have the potential to promote the use of written records so that the decision-making process can be more transparent. What they do not do, of course, is provide an answer or anything approaching an answer. In their notes accompanying the DECIDE model, Thompson et al. (2000) provide additional explication of each point. Under the heading 'Investigate Outcomes', part of the explication is the question 'What is the most ethical thing to do?', which is exactly the question that would originally have started the process. And this represents the main limitation of such models. They provide a context for thinking about the ethical issue but they still leave untouched the essential aspects of that issue to be perceived by the user and the core question(s).

Turning to models specifically developed for use by SLTs, we see that they tend to be similar in approach to the methods outlined above. For example, SPA has produced an *Ethics Education Package* (2002) that includes a decision-making protocol developed by Lamont and Brown (2001). This is based on five sections covering (a) the facts of the situation (such as who is involved), (b) the question of whether there is a problem requiring action, (c) a description of the problem in terms of ethical principles and duties, obligations or rules that are not being met, (d) a proposed decision and action plan, and (e) an evaluation plan.

The Consensus Model (Chabon & Morris, 2004), available on the ASHA website, has a similar structure. For example, where the SPA protocol queries whether there is a problem requiring action, the Consensus Model asks: 'Am I facing an ethical dilemma?', to be answered, say the authors, by checking whether the situation challenges personal and professional integrity. Similarly, where the SPA protocol prompts a description of the problem, the Consensus Model suggests that the nature of the dilemma should be stated clearly.

These two protocols have in common an emphasis on taking steps towards broader ethical reflection, rather than simply asking what is right or wrong in the situation. They also emphasise the need to gather all the facts of the situation and to determine whether the issue faced is in fact an ethical problem or some other sort of problem (e.g. a matter of personal preference or a legal matter). Further, both emphasise a consideration of multiple possible courses of action and evaluation of each of these. The Consensus Model highlights the need to examine a proposed course in relation to 'personal interests, social roles and expectations'. The role of the 'self' in ethical reasoning has been explored by Kinsella (2005). She suggests that professional discourses take precedence over the discourses of clients, and that this power imbalance can itself be an ethical issue (a theme we return to in Chapter 6). The Consensus Model therefore highlights the importance of thinking about whose perspective is considered and whose voice is attended to in ethical decision making. The flow diagram that accompanies the Consensus Model includes an iterative loop which divides around the issue of agreement as to the proposed course of action. If the course of action does lead to consensus, then the diagram suggests it is acceptable to proceed. If it does not, the diagram loops back into further analysis. Despite the apparent black-and-white nature of this dichotomy, Chabon and Morris dilute it by explaining that consensus 'is not 100% unanimity'. Clearly, ethical issues are such that often a complete consensus on appropriate action may not be achievable.

As with the approaches described earlier, protocols arising from speech and language therapy may offer a form of scaffolding to support consideration of ethical decisions but still leave the user with much to do in complex situations. They lend themselves to oversimplification of the process, risk encouraging underestimation of the complexity of the contexts in which decisions are to be made, and serve to exclude feeling and intuition from the process of making good ethical decisions.

We now turn to Seedhouse's (1998) ethical grid as an example of a somewhat different approach to making ethical decisions. The ethical grid consists of four concentric squares - referred to as layers - the inner three having four sections each and the outer layer having eight. The sections at the very centre of the grid represent the dual notions of 'creating autonomy' and 'respecting autonomy', together with the concepts of 'respecting persons equally' and 'serving needs first'. The next layer features duties such as keeping promises and telling the truth. The third layer focuses on the range of people potentially affected by the ethical issue - the patient, the decision-taker, a relevant group (e.g. 'children with cleft palate' or 'the Polish community') and society as a whole. Finally, the outer layer looks at external considerations – the law, available resources, risk, codes of practice, etc. Users of the grid are encouraged to start with whatever factors they feel stand out as most important and to use the various layers and sections to promote consideration of all relevant issues.

The grid is deeply grounded in moral philosophy – the second and third layers, for example, arise from strong ethical traditions relating to duty and consequences – and brings moral and societal factors out in a way that the step-by-step processes do not. It does, however, require users to understand the concepts they are dealing with, in particular to understand Seedhouse's central notions of creating and respecting autonomy and the relationship between them. Returning to SLT Alison's dilemma over the confidential information, these issues are certainly central. Although it may be tempting for the SLT to convey the information to other team members without risking the mother's refusal for such disclosure, Seedhouse would perhaps argue that there is a strong imperative to take action to create greater autonomy for the mother by giving her a chance to participate in the issue. At some point in this process Seedhouse's autonomy flip would take place and the question would move to respecting the mother's autonomous decision.

We have to recognise here that the issue of adults making decisions on behalf of children makes this much more complicated, since the mother's autonomy and the child's best interests (however these are defined) may be some distance apart. Baines (2008) has recently queried whether the concept of autonomy can legitimately be applied to young children at all and, if this is the case, whether the pre-eminence of the principle of autonomy in bioethical thinking is consequently doing all children a disservice. Such is healthcare ethics. This is another issue to which we return, in Chapter 6.

We have mentioned previously that a place for emotions, gut feeling and intuition is absent in our current constructs of good ethical decision making. As Mayeroff (1971) notes, wise decision making for practitioners engaged in relationships of care with clients may emerge from a mix of feeling and thinking. As SLTs we bring our individual experience and frames of reference to the ethical reasoning process. As a result, we need to develop 'good moral character' (Chabon & Morris, 2004). How we can develop this moral character to enhance our capacity to think and act ethically is the subject of the final section in this chapter.

Thinking ethically and being ethically proactive

An interesting exercise in teaching clinical ethics involves getting students or clinicians to write down a list of behaviours that they would see as constituting unethical conduct and then following this exercise with a description – and examples can be plucked from most people's personal experience with unsettling ease – of a health service interaction featuring what used to be called poor bedside manner. In other words, a situation where a health professional has interacted with brusqueness, dismissiveness or arrogance, without demonstrating that he or she understood someone's concerns and was committed to working to alleviate those concerns. Students and clinicians usually agree that poor bedside manner constitutes behaviour that is in some way not ethically good, but it is never on the list they have just written. This is presumably because it hovers just below a line of 'behaviour that is so ethically unacceptable we have to do something about it'. The problem with this entirely understandable position is that it leaves poor bedside manner as one of the numerous forms of interaction or behaviour that never reach the top of the agenda for consideration of their ethical ramifications.

What does it mean to practise ethically? Does it mean to follow the code of ethics of one's professional association? Does it mean to recognise ethical dilemmas when they arise in our work contexts and to act to resolve these dilemmas? Does it mean to pre-empt or avoid ethical dilemmas? Or does it mean to embed ethical thinking into our thought processes, our attitudes, our language and our interactions? It may not come as a surprise to learn that we think all of these have some place in our approach to speech and language therapy practice. Codes of ethics can provide a context for ethical thinking and a sign that a profession is at least aware of the importance of ethics, though, as we have discussed, they can serve to obscure the need for ongoing personal reflection. Ethical dilemmas undoubtedly occur in clinical practice and we need to learn to recognise them and have some strategies at our disposal for dealing with them. Ethical decision-making protocols can act as a starting point and a means of scaffolding these thought processes. But these are not – and will never be – enough. We need to learn to 'think and act ethically in ways that are deeply embedded in routine practice' (McAllister, 2006). Wright-St Clair and Seedhouse (2005) describe morality as 'a dynamic construction in the everyday, interactional world of human relating' (p. 18). The dynamic nature of this construction means that it requires constant, sensitive, flexible adjustment so as not to lose sight of the complexity of the 'commonplace matters of relating to and being with clients' (p. 19). This, according to Cribb and Duncan (2002),

> *requires us to be self-conscious about the values built into policies and practices, the different way in which our choices and actions impact upon others, the standards of conduct expected from people working in our occupational field, and the need to be able to explain and defend our practice to managers and clients. (p. vii)*

Recognising the fundamental moral nature of healthcare work involves what Seedhouse (1998) terms a paradigm shift. In practical terms the most important thing we can do is to bring discussion of ethics in speech and language therapy out into the open. This is not to say that ethical discussion doesn't take place in clinical practice now; in our experience it certainly does. But this discussion needs to be supplemented in two ways. Firstly the discussion needs to be recognised as being 'about ethics', and secondly it needs to come out from behind the closed clinic doors to be aired in public so that other people can hear about and contribute to it. To this end, the next six chapters throw open the doors of some areas of clinical practice to ethical scrutiny.

3 Dysphagia

Introduction

Asked to think of a situation in speech and language therapy practice that might present an ethical challenge, most students and many clinicians are likely to put dysphagia at or close to the top of their list. This is the field of speech and language therapy that touches closely the life-and-death, dramatic issues sometimes found in medical ethics. Patients can die if their clinical management is mishandled, and even the most theoretically safe and sensible clinical advice can be overridden by patients' views of their own quality of life. The aura of drama has accompanied dysphagia management throughout its development from a fringe area of speech and language therapy practice 25 years ago to its position as a cornerstone of the profession today. Some controversy was bound to accompany such a rapid move into the clinical spotlight.

Dysphagia has been defined as 'a delay in, or misdirection of, a fluid or solid food bolus as it moves from the mouth to the stomach' (Crary & Groher, 2003, p. 1). It generally refers to difficulty in any or all of the oral, pharyngeal or oesophageal phases of the swallowing process (though some definitions include sensory precursors to the motor process). A variety of conditions can give rise to dysphagia, some of which have acute onset (e.g. stroke) whereas others feature deterioration over time (e.g. progressive neurological diseases or tumours) (Logemann, 1998). Although dysphagia can affect any age group, our focus in this chapter is on adults.

Accurate figures for the number of people experiencing dysphagia are particularly difficult to establish, complicated by the variety of conditions involved and the associated differences in progression and recovery. As a rough estimate, figures given by Crary and Groher (2003) suggest that following stroke a high proportion (some 50%) of people experience dysphagia in the acute phase, with the percentage dropping towards single figures over the months after the stroke. Not surprisingly, the figures for progressive conditions increase with time and the same authors suggest that at least 50% of people with Parkinson's disease experience dysphagia at some stage of the disease. Specific subcategories of condition, e.g. the bulbar forms of motor neurone disease, have extremely high rates of dysphagia. Since dysphagia carries an inherent risk of aspiration (ingestion into the lungs of foods or fluids) and thus of respiratory complications, assessment has become imbued with a high degree of significance and often urgency. Various assessment techniques have emerged, ranging from identification of physical signs of swallowing difficulty via bedside assessment to instrumental procedures for viewing or hearing the swallowing mechanism in action, e.g. cervical auscultation, endoscopy and videofluoroscopy. A key challenge to all these procedures lies in the difficulty of identifying what constitutes a 'safe' level of aspiration. As noted by Sharp and Genesen (1996), 'the most common goal of intervention is to facilitate oral feeding using modifications in food texture, patient positioning, and/or the application of various swallowing techniques' (p. 15). When this is particularly problematic, the focus of management may move to non-oral feeding, with its own accompanying retinue of recommendations, decisions and management issues.

The question of how to assess dysphagia is accompanied by the question of who should undertake the assessment. SLTs have assumed a pivotal role in dysphagia work in general, but other health professionals such as nurses, physiotherapists and doctors could, in many cases, potentially be drafted in to the process. The challenge lies in untangling who has the skills and who has the time or opportunity to apply them. The resource allocation challenge across the professions is mirrored within speech and language therapy itself, exemplified (albeit simplistically) by competition for services in acute settings between people with dysphagia and those with communication disorders. This issue forms part of the backdrop to Scenario 3.1.

Scenario 3.1

Scenario 3.1 has as its setting an acute hospital where a junior doctor, a senior nurse, a newly qualified SLT and his manager are all considering the impending ward round. Central to their deliberations are two women: Mrs Banda, who has dysphagia (but is difficult to track down in her wanderings around the hospital), and the woman in the next bed, whose family are concerned about her communication.

Parvinder Singh, House Officer
10.30 a.m., Ward 16

Half an hour before the ward round. Parvinder mentally counts back – this is his eighth since qualifying and getting this job. He still feels the same lurch in his stomach that he had as a student when he thinks about ward rounds. Key things on his mind: Mrs Thomas – in the end bed – had a fall a couple of days ago trying to reach across to borrow a newspaper. She's been very subdued since then. The woman in Bed 2. It was difficult to make sense of what she was saying, though she sits and reads her newspaper so she must be reasonably OK. Mrs Banda in Bed 3. More often than not she wasn't actually anywhere near Bed 3 as she tended to wander about the ward and the nurses had to go and find her. As far as Parvinder could see, if Mrs Banda was well enough to be wandering about, she would probably be more comfortable wandering about in her own home or a nursing home or wherever. There was bound to be someone who could be making better use of the bed. He was pretty sure this was a view that would be expressed by Dr Giuliani at the ward round and Parvinder was keen to be get the situation sorted out beforehand. They always had to get the SLTs in to do a swallowing assessment, though Parvinder had wondered on occasion whether it wouldn't be easier just to do it himself. How complicated could it be? But Dr Giuliani was very pro speech and language therapy so that was that. Parvinder had seen Owen, the new therapist, coming onto the ward yesterday.

Owen Metcalfe, Newly Qualified Speech and Language Therapist
10.30 a.m., Ward 16

Half an hour before the ward round and he needs to get this dysphagia assessment finished. Except that Mrs Banda is nowhere to be found. Not only is the departmental target in jeopardy on this one but he needs the assessment results for the ward round. Owen is beginning to feel much more confident about these bedside assessments but there are a couple of things nagging him. He'd been quite taken with the technical side of videofluoroscopy during his degree studies but it seems almost impossible to get anyone referred for it. And then there's Mrs Banda. Well, not really Mrs Banda, though that's who they would all end up discussing again. It's the woman in the next bed (whose name, he is embarrassed to realise, he has temporarily forgotten) who makes him feel very uncomfortable. He managed 10 minutes with her a few days ago, got started on a screening assessment. She couldn't pick out any of the right pictures when he named them, though she gestured the right things. But he's had so many dysphagia referrals since then he hasn't managed to get back. He knows she's watching him when he walks past. And then yesterday, when he'd come down to do Mrs Banda's assessment, the daughter had demanded to know what he was intending to do to help her mother. She'd been very polite but she wasn't letting him go without information so he'd talked to her about aphasia instead of seeing Mrs Banda. Strange to think that if this woman started choking, she'd have to be seen. Mrs Banda hadn't been in her bed anyway. In the end he'd asked a nurse to do a dysphagia screening using the protocol he and Jackie had trained the nurses to use a few weeks ago for after-hours and weekend admissions.

Gloria Chin, Senior Nurse
10.30 a.m., Ward 16

Well he was certainly keen, the new speech and language therapist. He'd still been on the ward with Mrs Grace's daughter when her shift had ended last night and she'd come in this morning to find a note from him asking if the nursing staff could screen Mrs Banda's swallowing. Do these therapists think the nurses don't have enough to do already? Might have been better if he'd just got the swallowing assessment done himself and then they would be able to have a sensible discussion at the ward round.

Jackie Delaney, Senior Speech and Language Therapist
10.30 a.m., Speech and Language Therapy Department

She hopes Owen has managed to assess Mrs Banda because she knows what the consultant is going to say. Can Mrs Banda be discharged? We need to get her into somewhere more suitable.

She'd passed Owen in the corridor yesterday afternoon when he'd been looking for Mrs Banda. He'd given up trying to find her and asked the nursing staff to do the dysphagia screen. He also felt she needed to go for videofluoroscopy. Fine in theory but the clinic wasn't until Friday and Dr Guiliani was bound to say that Mrs Banda didn't want to be sitting around in hospital when she could come back for that as an outpatient. If Mrs Banda hasn't been assessed and can't be discharged, Jackie knows that Dr Guiliani will be on the phone straight after the ward round.

There had been a pretty frank exchange of views at the Stroke Services Management Group yesterday. Dr Guiliani had insisted that there was only one way they could meet waiting-list targets and that was for mobile patients to be discharged much more quickly. Dr Giuliani had always been fairly supportive of the speech and language therapy department but the hospital was in pretty dire financial straits and if they didn't hit the targets for this financial period, life was going to get a lot harder for all of them.

Commentary on Scenario 3.1

Rosemary Martino

This case scenario is a good demonstration of clinicians trying to achieve a balance between 'high-quality' care and 'efficient' care. Knowing how to strike this balance is not inherent and is rarely a quality of the newly graduated clinician. Let's take the example of Parvinder Singh and Owen Metcalfe, the former a junior doctor and the latter a speech-language pathologist. Parvinder and Owen have both recently graduated from their respective professional programs and are eager to apply their new clinical skills. At the same time, both are feeling pressured to meet the demands of hospital treatment and discharge protocols. As a result, the quality of care they provide to Mrs Banda suffers.

Parvinder's pressure stems from the need to reach a diagnosis regarding Mrs Banda's swallowing status. He is frustrated by having to wait for the speech-language pathologist to conduct this assessment. Parvinder is of the opinion that he himself should be able to assess Mrs Banda's swallowing ability. However, he feels 'forced' to a position of waiting because according to the unit protocols swallowing assessments are conducted by speech-language pathology. To further his frustration, he considers Mrs Banda ready for discharge because she is clearly able to ambulate independently around the ward. Hence, waiting for the swallowing assessment is delaying his ability to discharge Mrs Banda, free up a bed for a new patient and meet the hospital discharge targets.

In Parvinder's views, we see a simplified perspective of patient illness. In his opinion, a patient who can safely walk has no significant risk for dysphagia. Furthermore, Parvinder assumes he has swallowing expertise equal to that of the speech-language pathologist. He does not advocate for the collaborative team approach nor does he understand why Dr Giuliani (the senior doctor) doesn't recognize his ability to assess swallowing problems. Parvinder probably realizes that the presence of dysphagia can lead to serious consequences such as pneumonia, but it is clear that he underestimates the importance and the complexity of swallowing assessment. Parvinder has not yet learned the benefits of the team approach or the intricacies of the swallowing mechanics.

Interestingly, Owen's pressures also stem from the need to resolve Mrs Banda's swallowing status but from a different perspective than that of Parvinder. According to Owen, Mrs Banda's potential swallowing problems are not as interesting as the aphasia of the woman in Bed #2. Owen is frustrated by unit protocols, which require that he prioritize swallowing assessments over all others. Owen is further frustrated because whenever he comes by to assess Mrs Banda's swallowing, she is not in her bed. He considers scheduling her for a videofluoroscopy, but then decides to ask a previously trained unit nurse to administer a swallowing screening instead.

As with Parvinder, in Owen we see a limited perspective of patient illness – one according to his area of interest rather than patient symptoms. Owen, like many junior clinicians, is struggling with the ethical tension of sorting out how to allocate limited resources to dysphagia and aphasia. He is under pressure by virtue of his belief that the woman with aphasia in Bed #2 has a right to a service in the same way as Mrs Banda with dysphagia. Owen doesn't demonstrate awareness that unattended swallowing problems can lead to serious pulmonary and nutritional consequences. This is especially true in the acute medically unstable patient. For this reason, it is important to first establish if a swallowing problem exists and, if it does, establish at least some sort of compensatory plan that will ensure patient safety and reduce the likelihood of poor health consequences.

In this scenario, Mrs Banda has been identified as needing to have her swallowing assessed in detail. The purpose of a swallowing screening is to identify the presence or absence of a swallowing problem. Hence in a scenario such as this, where the presence of dysphagia appears to have already been identified, screening is of no added value. Gloria Chin, the unit nurse, is correct in her opinion that Owen is inappropriately delegating Mrs Banda's swallowing care to her. Instead, a full swallowing assessment by Owen is required to verify Mrs Banda's dysphagia, and, if present, to determine its severity, need for further assessment (such as videofluoroscopy) and appropriate treatment. Owen is clearly not aware of professional standards for swallowing practice that require completion of a full clinical assessment before videofluoroscopy. Determining the need for videofluoroscopy from clinical findings serves to refer only those patients who will likely benefit from this additional testing and thereby minimize both unnecessary healthcare costs and, more importantly, unnecessary radiation exposure for the patient.

Unlike Parvinder and Owen, Jackie Delaney (the senior speech-language pathologist) and Dr Giuliani demonstrate a more balanced focus between quality and efficiency of care. The pressure of meeting waiting-list targets has created a push for discharge of those patients who are ambulatory. This policy then places Mrs Banda, who is ambulatory, at high potential for discharge. Despite the current push for discharge, both Jackie and Dr Giuliani are advocating first for proper and timely assessment of Mrs Banda's swallowing status. The impression given in this scenario is that should Mrs Banda's swallowing assessment identify a serious impairment or a high risk for pulmonary or nutrition consequences, then proper follow-up and care will be secured before she is discharged. In this way, Mrs Banda is sure to get the best swallowing care in the most cost-effective manner.

In summary, this scenario highlights the need to mentor newly graduated clinicians in skills beyond those typically acquired during professional training. Both Parvinder and Owen inappropriately perceive the discharge protocols in isolation from quality of care. Greater awareness of Mrs Banda's situation by both Parvinder and Owen would allow (or indeed force) them to at least look outside their professional boundaries. Jackie Delaney and Dr Giuliani need to emphasize to these junior clinicians how Mrs Banda's care can be managed within these discharge protocols. One strategy, of course, would be to collaborate as a team. An informal discussion between Parvinder, Owen and nursing regarding the relative needs of the three patients in the same room might have generated a joint strategy on how to properly and efficiently assess all three before team rounds. For example, Gloria or Parvinder might have been able to update the daughter of the woman with aphasia in Bed #2 regarding her care, thereby freeing Owen to assess Mrs Banda's swallowing and possibly then also the aphasia of the woman in Bed #2. Gloria, rather than wasting her time screening Mrs Banda for a swallowing problem, could instead ensure that Mrs Banda is in her room when Owen comes by to assess her. Also, Owen could educate Parvinder on the dangers of dysphagia and its potential for poor health consequences even in patients who are ambulatory.

Both Parvinder and Owen appear well intentioned but are limited due to their modest clinical experience. It behooves those of us with many years of clinical practice to remember this limitation of those newly graduated. We need to take the time to teach them proper clinical judgment so that quality of care is kept in balance with efficiency.

Rosemary Martino, Assistant Professor, Graduate Department of Speech Language Pathology, University of Toronto & Affiliated Scientist, Health Care and Outcomes Research, Toronto Western Research Institute, Canada

Commentary on Scenario 3.1

Maggie-Lee Huckabee

Is non-optimal unethical? The question posed from this scenario very likely presents itself in similar circumstances in healthcare systems worldwide on a daily basis. It is a difficult question, and one that challenges the clinician and administrator to persistently adapt practice based on current research. The realm of dysphagia management is no longer in its infancy. We are moving quickly into a tumultuous adolescence with very rapid growth and perhaps awkward expansions into advanced clinical skills such as endoscopy, manometry, neuromuscular electrical stimulation and the like. Our rapidly expanding knowledge requires rapidly progressing clinical practices, but unfortunately this often must be done in a very slowly moving administrative system. In the scenario there are several issues that highlight substantive service delivery challenges which can undermine patient care and professional validity. As with all ethical issues, these are not easy to address.

We start this scenario with Parvinder Singh, juggling to balance patient needs with clearing beds. He doesn't seem to recognise the importance of speech and language therapy involvement in any of the patients. The patients from Beds 1 and 2 both appear with potential or demonstrated impairment of cognitive/language function; however, speech and language therapy involvement does not enter into his thinking. He is anxious to discharge Mrs Banda in Bed 3, based apparently on her ability to ambulate the ward, and sees swallowing assessment as just a box to tick off. He only hesitates in doing the assessment himself because he doesn't want to displease his superior. Very clearly the SLTs for this ward, either past or current, have not educated this emerging professional well regarding the complexities of swallowing physiology and the limitations of clinical assessment.

It's easily apparent why this is the case when we consider the behaviour of Owen, the current therapist. He is run off his feet and not getting his patients seen. He is struggling to balance dysphagia needs and aphasia needs, understanding that both deserve concentrated evaluation but having to prioritise in his very tight schedule. In most settings the emergence of dysphagia management into clinical practice did not come with an increase in clinical resources to manage an additional practice area. Thus, in this situation of having to choose between communication and dysphagia, Owen is acquiescing to the one that most imminently demands attention, in the form of an anxious family member.

Owen has learned about videofluoroscopic swallowing studies (VFSS) in his recently completed academic training, but is finding them infrequently done in clinical reality; bedside assessment seems to predominate, with little opportunity for diagnostic clarification. Are those in the academic ivory tower out of touch with clinical demands and not teaching to the 'reality' of clinical practice? Or are clinicians failing to advance their clinical practice to meet the minimum standards set by research? The American Speech-Language-Hearing Association (1992) published a position paper over a decade and a half ago that incorporated advanced diagnostic techniques into clinical work. Why are Owen and many clinicians like him still struggling to schedule VFSS? Finally, with his time and patience run out, he undermines his own professionalism by turning responsibility for swallowing assessment over to nursing staff. No wonder Parvinder thinks he can just do the swallowing assessment himself when the SLT minimises the value of his expertise in this way. Although there may well be a justified role for nursing screening of swallowing impairment in some populations, this should be a targeted programme, not a convenient solution when resources are stretched and the SLT doesn't have the time to do a proper clinical assessment. The senior nurse in the scenario, Gloria Chin, recognises this distinction and is not keen to undertake someone else's work.

The administrative demands of running a speech and language therapy department within the construct of a large healthcare system are many. Jackie Delaney, the senior SLT, is aware of this, but in her considerations of the issues in the scenario, she is diminishing one important variable: what the patient needs. Without a doubt, meeting financial targets is important; however, if this is accomplished by short-changing contribution to optimal patient care, little has been gained. In regions with a strong emphasis on third-party reimbursement, there is a growing trend to deny payment for 'bounce-back' admissions, i.e. patients who are discharged but quickly readmitted because healthcare needs were not adequately addressed during the initial hospitalisation. By report, aspiration pneumonia is a common aetiology necessitating bounce-back admission (Kind, Smith, Frytak & Finch, 2007). With consequences such as these on the horizon, an additional few days of hospitalisation to assure a careful assessment and well-thought-out plan becomes a much more financially viable option. Jackie notes that videofluoroscopy clinic is on Friday, several days away. Would it not be more beneficial from both a clinical and a financial perspective to negotiate with the departments involved to complete videofluoroscopic swallowing studies on an as-needed basis? Is this not another example, in many respects, of devaluing the contribution that is made through careful swallowing assessment? Diagnostic swallowing assessment must not be very important in the overall management of the patient if it can wait a week to be completed. Undoubtedly the radiology department has its own demands to address, but holding a patient on a ward or discharging prematurely and risking readmission while waiting for videofluoroscopy clinic is not an efficient use of time or resources. Another solution to this dilemma might be the incorporation of other diagnostic modalities, such as endoscopy, that can be completed without the scheduling restraints of VFSS. Although providing a different type of information than VFSS, this may offer sufficient insights into patient risks to allow interim progression of treatment planning.

The diagnosis and management of swallowing pathophysiology are proving much more complex than I think we ever expected in our early days of merging into this area of clinical practice. They present a substantive challenge to our academic and clinical training programmes, our clinical expertise and professionalism and the healthcare systems that either support or hinder our practices. Balancing patient, professional and administrative needs in this rapidly expanding area of practice inherently places the clinician on an ethical tightrope. Many individual clinicians and healthcare settings have risen to this challenge and maintained their footing. They address the complication of dysphagia with great expertise, employing carefully selected diagnostic and treatment procedures that are based on current literature. In these settings, service delivery programmes have asserted the importance of this area of practice by assuring that diagnostic procedures are scheduled as needed, the value of clinical services is undeniable when clinical and diagnostic precision support positive outcomes, and swallowing management is recognised by all healthcare workers as integral to patient outcomes for many diagnostic populations. In doing so, clear professional distinction is made and professional identity is respected and maintained.

Unfortunately many more clinicians and healthcare settings have not risen to this challenge and have consequently fallen off the tightrope. They continue to provide services that might have been acceptable 15 or even 20 years ago, but are clearly outdated based on current research. Although fiscal and administrative constraints may offer a short-term explanation while clinical practice adapts, it is not an acceptable long-term excuse. Substituting a quickly performed clinical assessment for the specificity of diagnostic examination because orders are too difficult to get is not only non-optimal, it is unethical. Substituting a nursing screening for a skilled clinical assessment because clinical services are under-resourced and not coping with the diverse needs of communication and swallowing is not only non-optimal, it is unethical. It is up to clinical services to advocate heartily for what is needed to provide optimal service to the patients in their care. By providing suboptimal care, a very real risk exists for undermining professional value, compromising patient outcomes and increasing long-term healthcare costs. Suboptimal is unethical.

Maggie-Lee Huckabee, Senior Lecturer, Department of Communication Disorders, The University of Canterbury & Van der Veer Institute for Parkinson's and Brain Research, New Zealand

Scenario 3.2

For Scenario 3.2 we move from the hospital setting to a long-stay care facility. The SLT and a family member have been in tense discussion about the advisability of non-oral feeding, and care staff are hovering in the background. Meanwhile, the man at the centre of the scenario is lying in bed, mentally compiling a list of favourite foods.

Strawberries probably.

Lisa, by now his favourite nurse, had had some strawberries in her bag the other night and she'd asked him if he wanted some. He'd only managed two, or maybe not even that. He'd spent most of the time trying to cough quietly.

Or roast potatoes.

Or possibly the cheese-and-onion sandwich he'd had on a ferry once when he hadn't eaten all day.

Maybe roast potatoes weren't quite the thing if there was going to be sand about.

Sometimes it was too unbearable to think about what you'd take with you to eat on a desert island, but then staying in bed all day and looking at four walls didn't have a lot going for it either.

For three months now he'd been in the nursing home, in a foreign world of immobility, stiffness and an endless round of toilets and bodily hygiene. Before he came into the home, he had been finding it harder to control his movements for several months and he had fallen a few times. In fact, it was only his daughter's input that had kept him semi-independent this long. They had both been concentrating so hard on him managing in his own home that neither had contemplated the possibility of a stroke as well. When your entire focus was on dealing with one illness, you developed an unexpressed expectation that you were immune from any other catastrophe.

Since coming into the home, he had become much weaker and there wasn't much left he could do for himself except think. Speech was getting harder to produce, and when he did make the effort, people seemed to have no idea what he was talking about. Sometimes he felt as if he had no idea what he was talking about either. Some of the staff had taken to talking to him in hushed tones, as if they were trying to get him off to sleep. It somehow made him feel both nurtured and alienated at the same time.

Patricia had brought the baby in to see him today. Not that she was so much of a baby any more, clambering over the bed and tugging at anything loose. Seeing her was the one thing that took him out of himself, took his thoughts away from the situation he found himself in. But when she had gone, it was like someone dowsing the only candle in a dark cell and he had to force himself to think about something else. Crying was too exhausting to contemplate.

Patricia had started up again about him having his food through a tube. He thought they'd already had this argument, though his side of it was generally more of an unspoken stubborn resistance. He was beginning to think that even Patricia only pretended to understand him.

'It just makes you cough, Dad, and then it'll go on to your lungs and you'll get really ill.' It did not seem possible to get much more really ill than he was already.

There had been raised voices – well, Patricia's raised voice – outside his room earlier on. He assumed it was the speech therapist getting some more advice from his daughter.

'He's supposed to be having his food pureed but I'm sure the staff are giving him other things to eat.' . . . 'You're supposed to be in charge of his food. Can't you get them under control?' . . . 'Anyway, he's going to have to be fed by tube because he can't manage anything else.' . . . 'I know you think that's not what he wants but you've only known him for three months.' . . . 'I've known him forever.'

As far as he could tell, the therapist was just trying to do a difficult job. She'd been quizzing him about food first thing this morning. It all came down to food these days. Or toilets.

'I wonder how a strawberry came to be under your bed,' she had asked. She must have eyes like an owl. 'Funny, I saw Lisa with some strawberries yesterday. I wonder if I need to have a word with her.' She looked at him intently as she spoke and he gazed inscrutably back. She picked the strawberry up off the floor and took it out of the room. He wondered hazily what she would have said if it had been a roast potato.

Commentary on Scenario 3.2

Maggie-Lee Huckabee

To feed or not to feed, that is the question – perpetually the question – in clinical management of swallowing impairment. Considerable time, effort and expense have gone into investigating the relative risks and benefits of oral feeding. And do we yet have the answer?

From a physiological point of view, no. We haven't tied down a clear answer to this question, despite considerable research. In our early years in dysphagia management, we asked the question 'How much aspiration is too much aspiration?', with the presumed belief that if we could answer this, we would be able to establish clear guidelines to resolve the feeding dilemma. There was great hope in the early 1990s that scintigraphy would be the tool to answer this question as it allowed for precise quantification of aspiration. However, when an answer seems simple, it inevitably is not. Firstly, scintigraphy is not widely available, is expensive and requires specialised nuclear medicine expertise, rendering it a not very practical solution. Secondly, and most importantly, the link between aspiration and pulmonary compromise is a bit like trying to pick up that elusive ball of mercury that has escaped a broken thermometer: the harder you grasp for an answer, the more indefinable it becomes. There is no clear cause and effect wherein if you eliminate the cause, you consequently eliminate the effect. The development of pulmonary symptoms requires contribution from a constellation of factors, which include such things as oral care, independence in feeding and resilience in pulmonary function, to name a few. Seminal research by Langmore and colleagues (2001) has given us substantial insight into risk factors and should be required reading by all clinicians. Although there are important caveats to their work, a key finding is that aspiration in itself it not sufficient to cause pneumonia. Thus, the question 'How much aspiration is too much aspiration?' becomes largely inadequate for addressing the decision of maintaining oral feeding.

But even if this question could be answered, clinical decision making is not simply an issue of physiology. The question of whether to feed or not to feed is equally influenced by quality of life. At its most basic, the ethical response to this question is quite simple: the patient has the right to choose his own course of treatment, including decisions regarding oral intake. It is the responsibility of the SLT, as well as others on the healthcare team, to provide thorough assessment appropriate to that patient's aetiology and presentation, and consequently place that information within the context of current research and current practice. It is not the role of the SLT to make patient choices or to feel responsible for the choices the patient chooses to make. Clinicians need to relinquish the paternal role in healthcare.

However, as with the physiological issues, the ethical issues are far from simple. Honouring patient choice is all well and good when patients are capable of processing information toward an informed decision and successfully communicating those choices to those involved in providing their care. In this scenario, we are provided with some insights into the thinking of the patient at hand; it's easy to assume that he might prefer continued oral intake. He thinks of food, or rather tries not to think of food. He savours the few tasty morsels that he receives despite the presumed discomfort and effort to inhibit outward signs of difficulty. He is exasperated with his daughter's persistence in discussing non-oral feeding and considers this a closed topic.

Unfortunately, clinical practice offers no clear insights into the internal cognitive processing and unexpressed desires of our patients. We have instead an abundance of patients who present with cognitive and/or communication impairment who are not able to indicate their understanding of the risk/benefit balance or articulate their desires for quality over quantity of life. The unfortunate man in this scenario exemplifies very well the imperative for evaluation and management of cognitive communication impairment as a component of swallowing assessment. In healthcare settings, there is a tendency for dysphagia management to take priority. We must recognise, however, the need to balance resources and not neglect this other area of practice that may direct swallowing management as substantially as biomechanical assessment.

Through the internal dialogue of this patient we see some coherence of thinking, recognition of his predicament and at least limited insight into risks. We also see desire and yearning for not only food, but also social engagement and understanding. Without this dialogue, or some compensatory mechanisms for communicating basic thoughts and needs (e.g. communication boards, written language or augmentative devices), we are left with imprecise and disputable interpretation of behaviour. Whether by the clinician or the family, determination of intent by behaviour is highly susceptible to bias and will ultimately represent the desires of the patient shrouded by the predispositions of the observer.

Consequently, clinicians often acquiesce to the requests of the family. Although undoubtedly the perceptions of the family will be biased by their own needs, in almost all cases the bias will be to the benefit of the patient. As this patient's daughter points out, 'I've known him forever'; she indeed may be in a better position to know what he would express if he were in a position to do so. But beware that not all family members may be capable of making those choices or may not use good judgement or good faith in reaching those decisions. Loved ones of patients don't always possess objectivity in their decision making and may not be able to extricate the patient's' desires from their own when they are experiencing the grief associated with potential loss of that loved one. On the more sinister side, I have been confronted in my career with a patient's family who insisted on continued oral feeding under the guise of improved quality of life. Careful scrutiny by a social worker actually yielded a much more selfish motivation in the form of a substantial insurance pay-out on the death of the patient. Although it is to be hoped that this represents the rare exception, it offers a reminder that context is critical in making decisions.

Frequently when students answer questions posed to them, my response is 'You're not wrong, but you're also not right', and there is something of this imprecision in the decision about whether to feed or not. At the far ends of the bell curve we will have clear and indisputable answers. More often we will have a clinical conundrum that challenges clinicians to look carefully at the effectiveness of both verbal and nonverbal communication, confer actively with patients and carers, and put aside their own preconceptions. Even then, the decision may be only slightly more right than it is wrong.

Maggie-Lee Huckabee, Senior Lecturer, Department of Communication Disorders, The University of Canterbury & Van der Veer Institute for Parkinson's and Brain Research, New Zealand

Commentary on Scenario 3.2

Rosemary Martino

This case scenario is a good example of the disparity among patient, caregiver and clinician opinion on what is most important – medical stability versus quality of life. The patient is a fragile gentleman who has dysphagia for solids secondary to stroke. He appears to have some functioning cognitive ability but with restricted communication and has dependency needs for his everyday care. He is now living in a chronic care facility and over time is getting weaker and more isolated. Fortunately, he has a supportive daughter who visits him frequently.

Although supportive, his daughter does not understand her father's refusal to have a feeding tube. She wants the feeding tube inserted so that his risks for developing pneumonia are reduced. The current evidence does not support this benefit of feeding tubes (Langmore, Skarupski, Park & Fries, 2002). In fact, if tubes are improperly managed, the frequency of pneumonia can be just as high with as without them. The daughter is likely not aware of the recent evidence and is naturally using her best judgment to advocate to maintain her father's good pulmonary health.

In contrast to his daughter, the patient's priority is his psychological health. Over time he is losing control over his basic bodily functions (such as walking and toileting) and his ability to communicate. He is increasingly becoming dependent and feeling more and more alone. In his isolation, he often thinks about the food he used to eat. He looks forward to the few treats of 'forbidden' solid food that the nurses sneak to him. These moments, along with the visits from his daughter and granddaughter, allow him to connect to his past life. They are the sparks that now keep him alive.

Also in this scenario are the speech-language pathologist and the nursing staff. The speech-language pathologist has accurately determined the risk for aspiration with solid foods. However, by reprimanding him for taking the solid food treats she runs the risk of making him feel even more isolated and with even less control. The nurses, on the other hand, are sympathetic to the patient's emotional state and, despite the recommendation by the speech-language pathologist, bring him a few treats here and there. In their opinion, what harm can a few treats really do?

In summary, this scenario has several players: the declining patient in a nursing home, his caring daughter, his competent speech-language pathologist and his emotionally caring nurses. This gentleman is fortunate to have these people in his life. However, he would have been even more fortunate if these people understood how his swallowing problem was affecting him psychologically.

The speech-language pathologist has a responsibility to competently assess the patient's swallowing ability (which she does), but also the responsibility to advocate on behalf of the patient and ensure that all decisions are made 'with' him and not 'for' him. Patient advocacy is especially important for patients like this gentleman who are limited in expressing their perspective because of cognitive and/or communication restrictions. The evidence shows that different people prioritize their health care related to dysphagia in different ways (Matino et al., in press). As in this case, clinicians and caregivers tend to prioritize the pulmonary consequences while patients instead prioritize their depression, isolation and dependency. The speech-language pathologist needs to be aware of this evidence and properly prioritize the patient's psychological health while managing his pulmonary and nutritional health. She needs to help the daughter understand her father's perspective and relate to her that feeding tubes will not necessarily provide the solution she was hoping for. Furthermore, the speech-language pathologist needs to help the nursing staff understand the severity of the patient's swallowing problem and his increased pulmonary risks for aspiration pneumonia and even death when they sneak in those solid food treats.

Together with the daughter, nursing staff and, most importantly, the patient, the speech-language pathologist will be in a better position to reach a diet texture recommendation that will best meet a compromise between the patient's desire for some control over his swallowing and the speech-language pathologist's and daughter's desire to reduce his risk for pneumonia. Also by being a part of this process, both the patient and the nursing staff will be more likely to support the recommendation.

In closing, this case scenario teaches us the reality of varying opinions among patients, their clinicians and their caregivers. What is important with regard to swallowing care depends on who you ask. This scenario also teaches us that as clinicians we must remember to address those factors most valued by our patients – the psychological issues – not necessarily as a substitute for that which we value clinically but instead (it is hoped) at a level of equal focus.

Rosemary Martino, Assistant Professor, Graduate Department of Speech Language Pathology, University of Toronto & Affiliated Scientist, Health Care and Outcomes Research, Toronto Western Research Institute, Canada

Discussion

As Martino says, when it comes to swallowing care – particularly where recommendations of non-oral feeding are concerned – what is deemed important depends on who you ask. Patients can and do refuse to go along with speech and language therapy recommendations. However well established a right to refuse may be, when the SLT is working in dysphagia, 'the practical implications of an actual refusal raise difficult questions for clinicians about their role in the face of such a refusal' (Sharp & Bryant, 2003, p. 287). Moreover, family and friends may disagree with patients, nurses may disagree with therapists, and so on. The situation becomes even more complicated when it involves adults who are not (definitively) competent to make decisions or whose wishes are difficult to discern. In this discussion, we look at the issues raised by disagreements over feeding in the light of the issues in Scenario 3.2. We then discuss issues related to the management of dysphagia in acute care arising from the differences of opinion on resource management in Scenario 3.1.

Although we as readers are privy to his thoughts, the wishes of the man in Scenario 3.2 in relation to oral or non-oral nutrition are not easy to discern for the other characters, a situation which has given rise to differences of opinion between his daughter, the SLT and the nurses. This in itself is inherently challenging, but the question of capacity to make the decision rests on essentially the same issues that questions of capacity raise across the board, namely whether the patient can understand and retain the information pertinent to this particular decision, weigh up the advantages and disadvantages of any proposed treatments and express consent or refusal. The significant underlying ethical question is ultimately whether the (competent adult) patient has a right to refuse treatment. A second, consequent question is what the SLT's options are if that is what the patient chooses to do.

Right to refuse

The right of competent adults to refuse medical treatment of any sort is, theoretically at least, well established by legal precedent in many countries. This precedent is based on the ethical concept of individual autonomy and also reinforces the weight accorded to it. Moreover, as Huckabee says, 'At its most basic, the ethical response to this question is quite simple: the patient has a right to choose his own course of treatment, including decisions regarding oral intake.' This legal right has been tested most publicly in circumstances where people refuse procedures that have obvious lifesaving potential, such as blood transfusion or amputation of gangrenous limbs, or procedures that will prolong life in circumstances of deteriorating or intolerable physical conditions, such as motor neurone disease. Such refusals are sometimes overtly based on religious belief, sometimes on a stated desire to die (and live) with dignity, and at other times on less clearly identifiable though no less firmly held personal values. But people refusing treatment are not generally held to be under any obligation to have 'good' reasons or in fact to explain their reasoning at all. To quote one example of the many expressions on this subject, Lord Donaldson in a UK legal judgment (Re: T [1992] 4 All ER 649) stated that a patient's right of refusal exists 'notwithstanding that the reasons for making the choice are rational, irrational, unknown or even non-existent'.

Although the right to refuse seems to be relatively straightforward, some of the underlying subtleties are evidenced by the fact that patients sometimes still have to resort to taking their cases to court despite supposedly not being required to give a reason for their decision. Once in court, their reasons for refusing treatment tend to be central to decisions about their competence to refuse. Stauch (2002) proposes that in practice 'the competent patient who refuses life-saving treatment for no reason may be a legal oxymoron' (p. 233); in other words, only 'incompetent' persons would refuse to have their life saved. Although this argument is primarily played out in the legal arena, the conundrum is relevant to the way in which the wishes of the man in Scenario 3.2 are interpreted. If he (by whatever means) refuses non-oral feeding, should the SLT consider overriding his decision in pursuit of his perceived best interests? To paraphrase Huckabee, the simple answer is no.

According to Tweeddale's (2002) view of doctors' reactions, cases where patients refuse treatment with serious consequences have the effect of revealing underlying paternalism. Tweeddale states that paternalism 'comes to the surface when doctors are asked by patients to follow a course of action which is in conflict with their own perspective' (p. 236). We should note that paternalism (setting aside the incongruous gender connotations of the term itself) may not simply be about health professionals thinking in some arrogant way that they know best, since recommending (from their perspective) the best treatment is what health professionals are supposed to do. Enforcing it, on the other hand, is not.

If the patient – as in Scenario 3.2 – refuses the SLT's best recommendation of non-oral nutrition, then the SLT's first ethical job is therefore to deal with any paternalistic instincts to override or undermine the patient's wishes. As Sharp and

Bryant (2003) say of decisions on feeding, 'to maintain true choice, nontreatment must be an option' (p. 290). The second clinical and ethical job is to consider how best to contribute to a course of action with which the SLT may fundamentally disagree, that is, how to actively help the patient to eat when the SLT doesn't think the patient should be doing so. As ever, this in itself may not be as black and white as it appears, since SLTs will be well aware of the pleasure and social importance that eating has for people, even if they are concerned by the physical consequences. As Huckabee says, 'it is not the role of the SLT . . . to feel responsible for the choices the patient chooses to make'.

Sharp and Bryant (2003) list some of the potential roles for the SLT in this position, including investigation of partial oral feeding, time-limited trials of therapy, and provision of information as to the safest method of eating within the limitations of the patient's physical status or, as Logemann (1998) puts it, providing the patient with 'information about the safest way to swallow within a range of nonsafe alternatives' (p. 364). The delicacy of this latter role is highlighted by the fact that Logemann further suggests that clinicians should write a report listing the alternatives but should not advocate a particular method. Taking this one step further, it is one of the few areas of speech and language therapy in which the literature actively raises the SLT's right not to continue to be involved, which we discuss in the next section.

Conscientious objection

Crary and Groher (2003) propose that 'the clinician has the right to sign off the case and pass it to another colleague who may have a different perspective' (p. 206). Although clearcut cases of SLTs opting out of particular clinical activities on the basis of their personal views may be relatively rare, the issue taps into a heated debate within medical ethics. It also resonates with questions about the extent to which the demands of professionalism require clinicians to put aside their own beliefs, values and in some cases emotions (an issue that is also discussed in Chapter 5). Lurking behind these issues, especially where dysphagia is concerned, may be the fear of litigation.

In medicine the issue of opting out is usually discussed in terms of certain medical treatments being against someone's 'conscience' or giving rise to conscientious objection. The most frequently debated contexts in which these terms arise are either at the beginning of life, e.g. birth control and abortion, or at the end, e.g. assisted dying. The issue in Scenario 3.2 might be thought of as just such a circumstance, in that it might be morally difficult for the SLT 'to participate in decisions not to do everything possible to prolong life' (Beauchamp & Childress, 2009, p. 42). The most common cause of such moral difficulty cited in the medical ethics literature, and the topic engendering the fiercest debate, is religious belief.

The tone of the debate, for the medical profession at least, can be gauged from Savulescu's (2006) assertion that 'if people are not prepared to offer legally permitted, efficient, and beneficial care to a patient because it conflicts with their values, they should not be doctors' (p. 294). His argument is that the determinants of medical care should be (a) the law, (b) just distribution of finite resources and (c) patients' informed desires, and that professionals' own values should not count as a determinant since these render healthcare inefficient, inequitable, inconsistent and discriminatory. Moreover, he argues that conscientious objection is incompatible with the commitment people take on when they become health professionals. On the other side of the debate is an argument that conscience is derived from an external (religious) authority (rather than from personal values), in addition to which Savulescu's use of the term 'beneficial care' is open to interpretation. An alternative way of viewing these opposing perspectives is that on the one side the integrity underlying a position of conscience might signal adherence to a strong and deeply held belief; on the other it might represent insistence that one's own values are simply more worthy than other people's.

Perhaps because this is an issue that is not seen to arise often, speech and language therapy codes of ethics do not specifically refer to a right to opt out, though they do encourage onward referral as necessary. The various speech and language therapy codes of ethics also refer in some form of words to the need for the welfare of patients to be held paramount. If the needs of a patient (as perceived by the patient) are in conflict with the views of the clinician, the word 'paramount' could be interpreted either as support for transferring care to someone else whose views might be in closer alignment with those of the patient or as obligation on the clinician simply to get on with the job.

Clashes of individual conscience and requirements of professional practice can often appear to be irreconcilable. Indeed, if the SLT in Scenario 3.2 holds a view that sanctity of life is more important than autonomous choice, it is difficult to see how she could contribute to advice on oral feeding. Lawrence and Curlin (2007) describe such questions as 'a debate that lacks middle ground' and conclude that 'recognizing disagreement and living with tension may be the only available avenue' (p. 13). Despite promoting a strong argument against health professionals being able to opt out of treatment, Savulescu (2006) offers two compromise positions. The first is essentially for such professionals to choose a different area of clinical work, where their conscience will not be challenged. The second is the suggestion that conscientious objection can be accommodated if it does not jeopardise the quality and efficiency of the clinical service. This, he says, requires that the number of professionals exercising the right to withdraw input remains below a critical threshold so that there are enough people to take on the work.

At the bedside of the man in Scenario 3.2, professionals and family members grapple with the ethical dilemmas and practical decisions of providing nutrition. The man in the middle of all this activity lies in his bed with no obvious means of expressing his thoughts in a way that will get them acted upon. It is not clear from the scenario how far the SLT has tried to help him establish a method for communicating or whether this is at all possible. Therein lies the issue to which we turn next. The balance between input to dysphagia and to communication impairment, here represented in a single person, occupies central ground in the current ethical life of speech and language therapy. To explore the issue further we focus in on the events in Scenario 3.1.

Dysphagia and communication impairment

In Scenario 3.1 we find ourselves in a busy hospital where staff are attempting to ensure that they are ready for the imminent ward discussion. This scene is played out in acute clinical settings every day, individuals rushing around trying to resolve questions of clinical management and deliberating how to make sure that each of their patients is treated (in all its meanings) well. It is worth just pausing to contemplate the complex undercurrents in such a situation. The state of knowledge about assessment and intervention in dysphagia is, as both commentators describe, not as clearcut as it might appear from a distance; all the staff have their own ideas about what is ethically fair and what is not; staff are at different stages in their development from 'newly qualified' to 'having the benefit of experience'; and into this volatile mix we can add the innate desire to maintain 'face' (and not to be seen to threaten that of others) in professionally challenging circumstances, with the constant interpersonal vigilance that such delicate negotiation requires.

'In most settings the emergence of dysphagia management into clinical practice did not come with an increase in clinical resources to manage an additional practice area.' (Huckabee). The resulting tension in acute settings between the demands of dysphagia work and the needs of people with communication impairments lends itself to some dramatic headlines: 'Are we eating our words?' (Balandin & Lincoln, 2003); 'Has aphasia been swallowed up?' (Enderby & Petheram, 2002). Although the discussion in this chapter arises from the setting of acute care and in relation to aphasia (which we will use as shorthand for communication impairment in general), it is an issue that concerns other areas of speech and language therapy. Balandin and Lincoln (2003), for example, focus on learning disability in all settings; Armstrong (2003) notes that the issues in acute care apply to people with dysarthria and dementia as well. In addition, as we have seen in the discussion of Scenario 3.2, it is not simply an issue of one population (with swallowing difficulty) in competition for resources with another (with communication difficulty), since the same person may present with both. It is an issue, though, of ethical importance both for the profession and for individual clinicians such as Owen who, 'like many junior clinicians, is struggling with the ethical tension of sorting out how to allocate limited resources to dysphagia and aphasia' (Martino).

The most obvious reason for the status shift of dysphagia work to a pre-eminent position in acute settings would appear to be the fact that it is primarily an acute problem. Aphasia, by contrast, is not. Dysphagia can be life-threatening, especially for people whose health is already compromised in some way. Aphasia, though it can have extreme consequences for a person's mental health, is not. The status of dysphagia in relation to these contrasting characteristics is perhaps the closest that speech and language therapy comes to the 'rule of rescue', an ethical concept from the field of resource allocation. The rule of rescue has its origins in 'the psychological imperative...to rescue identifiable individuals facing avoidable death, without giving too much thought to the opportunity cost of doing so' (McKie & Richardson, 2003, p. 2407). Although primarily focused on a societal preference for 'lifesaving over non-lifesaving measures' (McKie & Richardson, 2003, p. 2407), it also reflects the fact that 'people are generally prepared to extend very strong priority to the more severely ill at the expense of the less severely ill' (Nord, 1995, p. 207). Acute dysphagia work may not necessarily be a question of lifesaving or non-lifesaving measures, but the physical risks inherent in the management of swallowing may serve to foreground its rescue status. In addition, acute medical settings are predicated on rapid diagnosis and intervention and, if at all possible, cure. For professionals relatively unfamiliar with curative procedures, this may make it an inherently appealing area of work, however infrequently the 'cure' can actually be achieved. As Armstrong (2003) says, 'the possibility of assisting someone to return to a normal diet and resume normal eating patterns may well provide many speech pathologists with more satisfaction than working with individuals with ongoing lifelong difficulties' (p. 138). This is not to say, of course, that dysphagia has been accorded priority in acute care simply because it is potentially satisfying. In essence, it has taken priority because it is an acute problem and needs to be dealt with quickly. It would seem that SLTs, having developed skills in the area of dysphagia, now have an obligation to provide a rapid response for people with swallowing problems in settings designed exactly for that type of speed. The lack of ease with which people with aphasia fit the acute treatment system might be seen to place a different but equivalent obligation on the profession to meet this parallel need.

The design and function of acute healthcare settings are almost guaranteed to be an uncomfortable fit for people newly diagnosed with aphasia. Paradoxically, the experience of trying to adjust to the loss of communication ability amidst the commotion of acute care places the person with aphasia in a situation of similarly acute psychological need. Armstrong (2003) notes emerging evidence to suggest that although impairment-based therapy may be counterproductive in the early stages of such illness, approaches based on the facilitation of conversation are more promising. This is in addition to a seemingly obvious list of other types of assistance: accurate identification of what has happened, explanation to patients and family, charting of any progress, assistance with the functional requirements of communication in hospital.

Seedhouse (1998) describes an episode from his own experience of receiving healthcare for what turned out to be a benign lump in his cheek. To cut a long story short, he reports that the quality of care for his psychological needs fell a long way short of the quality of the intervention for his surgical needs. Seedhouse reflects on the significant distress he experienced as a result and suggests that this represented an ethical failure on the part of the staff:

> If the anaesthetist had failed to control my pain when it was within his power to do so then he would not have achieved a central goal of his work. Equally, and I insist on equally at this

point, if any health worker in any respect within his capabilities fails to control a person's pain in general when it is in his power to do so, he will have failed to achieve a fundamental goal. People suffer mental distress too. (p. 19)

Management and support of people with swallowing problems is now firmly established as one of the fundamental goals of speech and language therapy in acute settings. Previously it was also the case that development and maintenance of what Armstrong (2003) terms a good 'communication culture' in acute settings was also seen as a fundamental goal. It is difficult to see an ethical argument to suggest that this should somehow have changed.

Summary

SLTs working in dysphagia may find themselves at the interface between two very different worlds: one based firmly on the medical model and the other, encompassing many of their fellow speech and language therapy colleagues, leaning in many instances towards social integrationist models of healthcare. As such, dysphagia work raises dilemmas familiar to medical ethicists, such as refusal of treatment (with potentially serious consequences), and also issues of focus and resource allocation within the profession of speech and language therapy. In addition, despite the firm foundation that dysphagia work now has, boundaries and workload responsibilities between SLTs and other professions are still being negotiated.

The right of adults to refuse treatment is superficially straightforward and can legitimately override even the most earnest clinical advice. But as we have seen, in practice the right to refuse non-oral nutrition can be complicated by competing family interests, difficulty in establishing safe levels of aspiration and difficulty in ensuring that patients can make and express autonomous decisions. Furthermore, faced with a refusal of non-oral feeding, SLTs may find themselves working towards a goal they fundamentally disagree with or exploring the possibility of opting out.

Workload and caseload pressures in acute settings lend themselves to prioritisation of the most urgent physical needs, as do well-established ethical obligations in relation to lifesaving treatment. This pressure seems unlikely to decrease in the near future. At the same time, the needs of communicatively impaired people in acute settings have not changed substantially during the time that dysphagia work has been developing. The ethical obligation to meet those needs has not changed substantially either.

4 Intellectual and sensory impairments

Introduction

In this chapter we discuss ethical issues that can arise in SLTs' work with people who have intellectual and sensory impairments. The scenarios in the chapter attempt to capture some of the nuances of practice with both adults and children with disabilities. The focus is on intellectual and hearing impairments, though many of the issues captured here apply also to people with congenital motor impairments (such as cerebral palsy) and visual impairments. We have chosen to focus on intellectual impairments and hearing loss because people with these impairments appear in generalist speech and language therapy caseloads.

Definition of intellectual impairment is sometimes expressed in terms of IQ (i.e. equal to or less than 70), but a government report by the Scottish Executive (2000, p. 3) provides a more straightforward – and sensitive – functional definition (of what they term learning disability).

> People with learning disabilities have a significant, lifelong condition that started before adulthood, that affected their development and which means they need help to:
>
> - understand information;
> - learn skills; and
> - cope independently.

The clarity of this definition is not quite matched by the terminology, where learning difficulty, learning disability, intellectual disability and intellectual impairment are all in use. The Scottish Executive report notes the increasing use of 'intellectual', in preference to 'learning', and this has been standard practice in other countries for some time.

The same report estimates the prevalence of mild or moderate intellectual impairment to be 20 people in 1000, with three or four people in 1000 having profound or multiple disability. Language, speech, voice, fluency and swallowing impairments can all co-occur with intellectual impairment.

Many people with intellectual impairment will benefit from some form of augmentative or alternative communication (AAC) (Beukelman & Mirenda, 2005).

This may be low-tech AAC such as signs or picture/symbol boards, or high-tech such as computerised voice synthesisers or word processing software. SLTs are often involved in recommending and trialling AAC systems and in training people with disabilities, their families, teachers and carers to use the selected systems.

Working with people with long-term disabilities is different from much of speech and language therapy practice in that SLTs may be involved over a long period of time, possibly from the client's infancy onwards. Services for people with disabilities are often multidisciplinary in nature and require regular interaction between team members. SLTs may therefore come to know the person, the family, the carers and other involved professionals very well. They may develop significant relationships with the person and the family, as opposed to the caring but nonetheless professionally distanced relationships that are more typical of short-term clinical interaction. As skilled and empathic communicators, SLTs may be involved in communication with families about highly personal and sensitive matters. Further, as skilled users of low- and high-tech AAC, they may belong to a very restricted set of people with whom an AAC user can communicate at a deep level. The SLT may therefore become privy to information that is not only confidential but possibly also controversial and confronting. The potential benefits and drawbacks of this type of relationship come to the fore in both our scenarios.

Medical advances such as immunisation for rubella and genetic screening have led to a decrease in the incidence of congenital sensorineural hearing loss (Ries, 1994). Universal newborn screening is leading to earlier detection and fitting of hearing aids for children (Northern & Downs, 2002), and an increasing number of hearing families are choosing cochlear implants for their children with severe-profound sensorineural hearing loss. Some deaf parents are also opting for cochlear implants for their children, inflaming the long-running debate about the merits of cochlear implantation and its impact on Deaf culture (see, e.g., the US National Association of the Deaf policy statement [2000] on cochlear implantation).

Habilitation and speech therapy for children post-implantation have until recently followed an almost exclusively auditory-verbal approach, without use of visual cues derived from facial expressions and lipreading. More recently, therapy approaches which allow the child to use both auditory and visual cues after implantation have been employed in some centres (Christiansen & Leigh, 2004; Swanwick & Tsverik, 2007).

Families who choose cochlear implantation face a long engagement with spe-cialist cochlear implant teams for pre-surgical assessments, post-implantation monitoring and extensive habilitation. As these cochlear implant teams tend to be based in major cities, families from smaller urban centres or rural areas may face extensive travel, with associated costs and disruptions to family routines. Although early habilitation post-implantation is typically done in specialist centres, families are often referred back to SLTs in their local communities for long-term speech and language therapy. SLTs in a range of paediatric service settings may therefore find themselves with children with hearing loss on their caseloads, and it is to such a situation that we turn for our first scenario (Scenario 4.1).

Scenario 4.1

This scenario illustrates the difficult decisions faced by many parents considering a cochlear implant for their child. Anthea is the mother of Poppy, who has a significant hearing loss and for whom cohclear implantation has been recommended. Anthea is seeking assistance in her decision making from SLT Susan.

'What would you do if Poppy was your daughter?'

Anthea posed the question, sat back in her chair and held Susan's gaze. Susan's stomach lurched; she'd asked herself this question hypothetically during both her pregnancies. Years ago as a new graduate she'd worked in a school for the deaf that used total communication, and later she'd been employed in a cochlear implant (CI) centre. Having a child with a hearing loss was something that had been on her mind, but, as it turned out, both her children had normal hearing.

Susan already knew Anthea and her husband, Peter, before they came to the clinic with Poppy. They had a son, Dylan, who had a significant intellectual impairment and communication and behavioural problems. As the only SLT in this country town, Susan had provided blocks of speech therapy to Dylan and worked with the psychologist and parents on behaviour management strategies. Susan's youngest child had attended the same preschool as Dylan, and Susan and Anthea had come to know each other a little while waiting to collect their children at the end of the preschool day.

Dylan had gone off Susan's radar since he started school; he was now managed by the education SLT service. She had been shocked to receive a referral from the local GP three months ago to see Peter and Anthea and their year-old daughter, Poppy. The GP suspected Poppy might have a hearing loss and had also referred the family for audiological assessment. The audiologist had found a severe hearing loss and had talked to Anthea and Peter about options for Poppy. One of those was cochlear implantation. Peter and Anthea had visited the CI centre in the city, a three-hour drive away.

Peter and Anthea made this appointment to see Susan to discuss treatment options for Poppy. The CI centre had told them that Poppy was a suitable candidate for a CI. Although the parents believed that Poppy would benefit from a CI, they were very concerned about the follow-up commitments expected of them. They had been told that by agreeing to an implant, they were also agreeing to bring Poppy for weekly follow-up and therapy sessions for a year. Anthea would be able to drive Poppy to the city for therapy each week, but they were worried about how they would cope with the long day or possible overnight stay and the home practice the CI centre demanded between visits, given their son's needs and their tightened budget. Anthea gave up paid work when Poppy was born. 'Just as well I did really because Dylan is still so hard to handle – he takes up so much of my time and I am up at the school most days.'

In addition, Peter and Anthea were disturbed by conversations they had had with some deaf adults who attend their church with their deaf teenage children. 'They told us we had no right to decide for Poppy that she would have a cochlear implant,' Anthea said, 'and that if we did, we would be cutting her off from the deaf community in the future, because she won't learn to sign.' 'We're damned if we do and damned if we don't get this implant' Peter said.

Susan now found herself frantically thinking how to respond to Anthea's question. What *would* she do if this was her daughter, given her ambivalence towards the strict auditory-verbal approach used in post-implantation (re)habilitation in the city? She had concerns over the fact that the auditory-verbal approach used at the centre excluded the use of visual cues to help implanted children discriminate speech. It seemed to her to fly in the face of all she knew about the role of nonverbals in normal communication. She was half-inclined to be frank about her concerns, but that might dissuade them from making what could ultimately be a good decision for Poppy. On the other hand she knew that if Poppy did not have the CI and stayed here, she was going to need lots of input. Susan just didn't know how she'd manage to fit that in.

Meanwhile, Anthea waited calmly for an answer.

Commentary on Scenario 4.1

Sandra Van Dort

I can empathize with Susan's trepidation at having to discuss treatment options for Poppy. The dilemma the parents face is a real one in the sense that whatever decision is made, costs for Poppy, her brother Dylan and the family seem inevitable.

In one sense Poppy has a right to the better audition that a cochlear implant will bring. The CI team has confirmed the appropriacy of her candidacy. She is one year old, and thus the potential to gain better access to the spoken language signal, when coupled with early intensive intervention, will significantly impact on her verbal language acquisition.

However, in another sense, one cannot ignore the fact that Poppy is a deaf child, and although the CI is a tool that can provide access to better hearing, it cannot cure her condition. She should then also have a right to early access to sign language and communication with the deaf community, and this relates to the psycho-social aspect of her development. The comment by the family's deaf church friends that Poppy may be cut off from the deaf community because she hadn't learned to sign is a case in point. The auditory-verbal approach used at the CI centre may be an approach that excludes the use of any visual cues and signs.

The second issue that arises out of this situation is the burden of care the family is faced with, in terms of personal energy, finance and time costs. Given the needs of their other child, Dylan, the additional commitment and costs of the CI programme will strain an already strained system. In my own practice, I have seen parents withdraw from the CI programme offered at our local clinic after the pre-operative interview. Aside from collecting funds to cover the implant and habilitation costs, parents have to commit to weekly appointments and intensive habilitation. For many families who are not affluent or who live some distance away, these resources are simply unavailable. Hence this second problem, a CI programme that does not appear to have made accommodation for family needs, is another ethical issue to be considered.

The third issue is the fact that the parents in this scenario have not been given enough information to make a decision that is informed. I would assume that most CI programmes will do an adequate job of counselling parents about the potential medical risks and benefits of a CI and perhaps even have discussed appropriate expectations for communication outcomes after implantation. However, this CI programme appears not to have provided the parents with an understanding of other communication options. These parents have instead got this information from their church friends, but it has not been presented objectively. Indeed, the parents appear to have been accused of 'damaging' Poppy if they decide on implantation.

The final issue is that the therapist, Susan, has acknowledged some biases, namely her professional uneasiness with the auditory-verbal approach based on her working experience and theory. Further, she is also faced with the dilemma that if the parents decide on hearing aids instead, she would have the job of providing intensive intervention for Poppy and is unsure of being able to do this.

What should be done?

I would think firstly that Susan must not respond directly to Andrea and Peter's question. Rather than influencing parental decisions by offering a personal opinion or bias, it would be more important perhaps to interpret the inferential content of that question back to the parents, acknowledging the fact that the parents are having enormous difficulties coming to a decision and are seeking help. Susan could then suggest some strategies the parents could use to reach an informed decision.

One strategy, as mentioned above, would be to address the dilemma the parents face over the rights of Poppy to amplification versus Deaf culture identity. Given that Poppy is too young to make her own decision, it is ethically correct that her parents make this decision for her. The fact that Poppy's parents are hearing parents will also weigh on the decision they make. However, more comprehensive information about benefits and costs needs to be gathered. Indeed, the use of either a CI or high-powered hearing aids, combined with an intensive intervention programme with an oral emphasis, would benefit Poppy in terms of providing her access to the hearing world. Conversely, the presence of the deaf family in the community would be an excellent resource, if the parents opted for a visual communication system. The positive and negative benefits of each approach should be clearly evident for the parents, so that they can make an informed decision. Further, even if the parents decide on implantation, access to signing and interaction with their deaf family friends should be made available when possible and it should not be perceived in an all-or-nothing way. The parents also need to be given comprehensive information from Susan about the intervention programme that she could realistically run for Poppy, if they decided against implantation but for a hearing aid fitting.

The second issue is much harder to resolve. It is partly a result of current service delivery characteristics that encumber families with limited resources. Firstly, it must be stated that the CI is an expensive device and that the rehabilitation related to it is also expensive for many families, in terms of commitment, finance and time. For instance, CI programmes are usually run in major cities and along traditional protocols that demand sacrifices of time and money. Service delivery options that accommodate all types of families should become a standard feature of such programmes. This is an ethical issue of service delivery that we as professionals should strive for (Hyde & Power, 2006) and every effort should be made by the CI team to allow for this, if the parents go ahead with implantation.

It is also important for Susan to make clear to the parents that once they have better knowledge of the issues, whichever option they choose can be a viable option for their child. Choosing to forgo a CI or hearing aid for a child with severe to profound hearing impairment is legal in Malaysia, for instance. However, the parents must be aware of the implications of this decision for their child.

Susan's role would thus be to enquire and ensure that the parents had the knowledge necessary to make an informed decision about their child. If she did not have the information, Susan could refer parents on to obtain it, perhaps from the CI team or from the local deaf persons' organisation. Finally, her previous interactions with the family and her role with their first child make her ideal as a person who could provide some emotional support for both parents and bolster parent confidence, in order that that they make their best decision for Poppy and the family.

Sandra Van Dort, Senior Lecturer, Department of Audiology and Speech Sciences, Faculty of Allied Health Sciences, Universiti Kebangsaan Malaysia

Commentary on Scenario 4.1

Loraine Fordham

What would I do if Poppy was my daughter?

That a parent should cause us to ponder this question is understandable. Don't we ask similar questions to 'friends in the business'? Working over time in any specialised field of speech pathology, we develop expert knowledge about the range of therapeutic outcomes, as well as an understanding of what factors work for and against those outcomes. It can be very tempting to give a quick one- or two-sentence answer to such a question, because I know what I would do if faced with this dilemma. But...Poppy is not my daughter, or Susan's daughter, or any other SLT's daughter, and so irrespective of any biases we have about therapeutic options, it is not our role to direct or influence a family's choice.

Additionally, questions related to paediatric cochlear implantation are possibly some of the trickiest to ponder. There are conflicting, emotive issues that require resolving, and in this family's case there are compounding factors.

What are some of the key issues to take into account?

Firstly, cochlear implantation is not a quick fix. It requires an enormous amount of work by the family, who must attend therapy sessions in order to learn how to implement therapeutic goals functionally in their child's natural environments. But this family lives far from where the rehabilitation program is located, and there will be huge demands on the parents' time, as either both parents (the ideal situation) or one parent will regularly attend therapy sessions.

This will involve making adjustments to their daily routine: managing the time away (at least a day a week) and the extra finances required (petrol definitely but possibly overnight accommodation). They will need emotional support and personal resilience as they commit to learning new therapy techniques. They will also have to balance any decisions or actions they take for their daughter with what those will mean for their son. For example, does he tag along every week, or will they need to find and budget for a carer to mind him?

In addition, some parents are understandably nervous about the type of surgery involved, as the procedure involves the child's head (often an emotional aspect) and families require support and counselling both before and after the procedure.

Secondly, there is the perspective of the Deaf community, whose views these parents have already experienced. The Deaf community disapproves of paediatric cochlear implantation, believing that it denies a deaf child access to their rightful deaf culture and language. It believes parents should not take this decision for their child, but that either the child should be involved in the decision process, or that parents should choose sign language until the child becomes adult and can make up his or her own mind. The Deaf community also correctly argues that implantation destroys the residual hearing of the implanted ear, which means there is no chance of retrieving that hearing if in the future further technological advancements surpass implantation.

However, the majority of deaf children are born to hearing parents, and this factor is often the most salient for hearing parents. They ask themselves, 'How will we communicate effectively or fluently with our deaf child?' or 'How will our child function in a hearing world?' Most influentially, there is now a growing body of international research to show that with intensive early intervention, profoundly deaf children who are implanted in their early months can develop very good listening, speech and language skills.

Be that as it may, whatever option they choose, this family will require support from their local SLT. Unfortunately if the parents choose implantation, this SLT is not totally supportive of the auditory-verbal therapy approach. And should they choose hearing aids or sign language or a combination of both, she would not be able to provide the extensive therapy that Poppy would need.

How to proceed?

From my experience, I would tell these parents that while I cannot answer their question directly (because only they know what will be best for their child and their family), I will nonetheless be a supportive, collaborative partner in their decision-making process. Steps to achieving this are outlined below.

Steps in the collaborative decision-making process

Clarify whose decision this is

Support families by suggesting ways they can increase their knowledge and confidence in making their decision. In light of the disparity between the medical and the Deaf community's perspectives on paediatric cochlear implantation, it would be important to provide this family with credible sources of information that assist their understanding of both views, while reinforcing whose decision this is.

Clarify the intervention choices and the likely consequences of each choice

In this scenario there are three options to consider:

* *Cochlear implantation*: This might involve pre-implant assessment and training sessions before implant surgery, followed by intensive auditory-verbal therapy. For Poppy to maximise the benefit of her implant and to achieve good listening,

speech and language skills, she will require regular therapy well beyond a year. This fact must be made clear to the family beforehand.

▨ *Hearing aids*: Poppy could be fitted with bilateral hearing aids, after which she would need regular/intensive speech and language therapy to achieve good listening, speech and language skills. She would require regular paediatric audiology services to monitor her hearing levels, and to monitor and adjust her hearing aids accordingly.

▨ *Signing*: Poppy and her family would need intensive sign language training and they would need to find educational settings that support Poppy's communication style.

Help families get the best information

To make the best decisions, families need the best information. It is a good idea to ask families what type of information they like:

▨ Do they like written information, such as fact sheets or textbooks?
▨ Are they confident using the internet and can they evaluate Web resources?
▨ Do they prefer talking to people face-to-face or over the phone?
▨ Do they like to see things in action?

Families may be comfortable with all the above methods or they may prefer one or two. Taking an eclectic information mix, I would recommend the following:

▨ Talk to the implant centre to find out if there is another audiological assessment that could provide additional information to help this decision.
▨ Encourage these parents to talk to other parents who have experienced a similar decision-making process.
▨ Provide contact details of diverse early childhood intervention programs for deaf children, e.g. an auditory-verbal program, a total communication program, a signing program and/or preschool.
▨ Encourage the parents to visit these centres, to observe the children and meet the teachers in the different settings.
▨ Establish what rural networks exist to support this family.
▨ Find out what training courses exist for families and SLTs in both auditory-verbal therapy and signing. Explore residential options.
▨ Identify credible websites representing the Deaf community, hearing aid services and the auditory-verbal approach.
▨ Source recent journal articles that compare children with CIs, children with hearing aids, and children who sign across a range of outcomes.
▨ Source articles by parents who have been through similar circumstances.

Help families to evaluate and select the intervention that will best meet their child's and family's goals.

Loraine Fordham, Speech and Language Pathologist & Doctoral Student, Institute of Early Childhood, Macquarie University, Australia

Scenario 4.2

The scenario below presents a sadly all too common situation in residential care for people with disabilities, that of communication breakdown between carers, therapists and clients. Kieran, an adult male in a group home, has disclosed sensitive but ambiguous information to his SLT, Andrew, which calls for tactful action by Andrew.

'Are you sure he called them that?' asked Bill, Andrew's Team Leader.

'Well, Kieran doesn't speak at all, but he's a very good Makaton signer, got a huge vocabulary, signs clearly,' replied Andrew, 'and he's got a very expressive face. Plus, I've been the SLT visiting that group home for years. I know Kieran pretty well.'

'I suppose that might explain why he would tell you and not the care workers,' said Bill.

'Yes. He told me because he trusts me, I suppose. I can sign as well as he can. I've always laughed at his jokes and I've never stopped him talking about girlfriends. He might have Down Syndrome, but that doesn't stop him wanting to live an adult life and he *is* 28 after all. He asks me to help him find a girlfriend almost every time I go to the home,' said Andrew, 'but last week there was something different about it. Kieran can often be quite – um – negative in the way he describes his care workers and I can see why. They're pretty jaded with the whole setup – short-staffed, underpaid. They've lost interest in training and I've given up trying to get them to brush up on their signing. The end result is that they restrict Kieran's independence because it's too much like hard work to facilitate it. So apart from going to the shop to fetch milk and the occasional trip into town, he's confined to barracks.'

This was not a happy situation and it looked set to get worse.

Last week on Andrew's visit to the group home, Kieran had started signing about having sex. This was where the efficiency of signing as a medium came distinctly unstuck. Although Kieran was very animated in his communication, by the end it was still not clear to Andrew if Kieran was indicating that he had already had sex with someone or that his need to have sex had reached some sort of critical level. Either way, the warning lights had started flashing in the Risk Assessment Section in Andrew's brain. If Kieran had already started a sexual relationship, who was it with? Another resident? Someone in the community who Kieran had met? (And if it was the latter, how on earth had he managed that?) Consensual? Safe? Birth control? Adjectives and nouns started going off in Andrew's head like fireworks. What if Kieran wanted the care workers to arrange a visit from a sex worker? Or *to* one?

Andrew had asked Kieran if he had told the care workers. Kieran had shrugged and signed something very clear and very rude. Andrew had tried to raise his concerns with one of the care workers in the kitchen, but had met with a dismissive response.

'Yeah right; like that's going to happen.'

'But we've got to take this seriously. Kieran's health and safety might be at stake. And somebody else's.'

Andrew was taken aback by the vehemence of the care worker's response.

'Look, it's all under control. And anyway, is it you that's going to be there to pick up the pieces when it all goes wrong? No, of course it isn't. You need to remember you're a speech therapist and not a bloody social worker.'

Commentary on Scenario 4.2

Celia Harding

Summary of key issues

Andrew is a speech and language therapist who works with adults with learning disabilities. He has raised an issue of concern with his line manager, Bill. This has involved one of his clients, Kieran, who has wanted to discuss sex. In Andrew's view he has never stopped him talking about girlfriends. It is not exactly clear what Kieran wants to discuss about sex, but we are aware that he has expressed it through Makaton.

Kieran is an adult with an intellectual impairment who has developed a positive relationship with Andrew. He has been supported in learning and developing more adult Makaton signs suited to his needs. However, an issue has arisen about understanding what Kieran is communicating. Kieran has a basic vocabulary to discuss sex but his usage is limited and therefore this puts him at risk of being misinterpreted; it is not clear if Kieran has had sex, and if so, who with? Andrew rightly assumes that there could be a significant risk issue here, principally in terms of Kieran's health.

Andrew has made an assumption that the care workers feel undervalued in their job, and has interpreted this as having an impact on their motivation to support their clients effectively. Andrew's views about the care workers are that 'They're pretty jaded with the whole setup – short-staffed, underpaid. They've lost interest in training.' There is an issue with the care workers, but their voice has not been given enough profile for us to reflect on what their views actually are. The care workers' opinion is not really expressed in this scenario until the end: 'You need to remember you're a speech therapist and not a bloody social worker.' The same care worker expresses the opinion that the issue Andrew has raised on Kieran's behalf is 'all under control'. Further, in the difficult exchange about this issue, the care worker expresses the view that Kieran having sex is very unlikely to happen. Finally, should Andrew be actually discussing with his manager his concerns about Kieran and the care workers without other relevant professionals present?

Why the issues present challenges

Andrew appears to be passionate about adults with intellectual impairments having full access to their rights. It seems as if he has taken on this mantle of responsibility as part of the remit of his job. This an issue that requires a more careful multidisciplinary team approach, and also where Andrew needs to be considering Kieran's level of communication competence. Kiernan's rights need to be respected and valued by all who work with him. However, there needs to be a realistic understanding of his needs using a person-centred planning approach. This would have to involve an advocate as it appears that people are interpreting Kieran's needs from their individual perspectives, perhaps because they feel he has a right to access something regardless of the wider issues involved. Staff seem to have placed their own interpretations on the issue at hand and reacted, rather than discussing the issues more formally within the multidisciplinary team.

There are many elements of risk highlighted within this scenario, and these all present challenges. For reasons not clear, the care workers lack motivation to maintain or improve their signing, thereby putting themselves at risk of inadequate communication with their clients. Consequently, Kieran is at risk of having his needs misinterpreted by people who should be supporting him and making informed decisions with him or on behalf of him.

How the issues might have arisen

Poor communication and lack of motivation within the team have meant they have reacted to a 'problem' rather than working cooperatively in a proactive fashion to anticipate and prepare for such a situation. There is a worrying lack of involvement of other professionals within this scenario, such as consultants, care staff, advocates, health care workers, social workers, and so on. It is also possible that Andrew's view of the care staff as unmotivated has led him to not engage fully with them and make clear Kieran's communicative capacities and needs.

Bill may need to reflect on his management of Andrew. Are his support and supervision productive, with appropriate goals, or are the meetings filled with similar sorts of issues? It may be that Bill is not clear about the issues involved when working with people who use augmentative and alternative communication, and the risks that can arise from misinterpretation of clients' communications.

Alternative and proactive approaches to managing this scenario

When working with people who have complex communication needs, goal planning needs to be within a team context. SLTs are often the key professionals whom people with communication disorders feel most comfortable talking to about their problems and difficulties. This is inevitable as the SLT understands in more detail the nature of the communication difficulties, how to facilitate and promote communication, and has a clear idea of the receptive function of the client. This is acknowledged by many other professional groups. Interpretation of communication by people who use augmentative and alternative communication always requires careful goal setting in collaboration with key people who work with service users. Consequently, the rationale for the system needs to be fully understood by all involved, including the service user. Can the service user understand the system and have the vocabulary relevant to his or her needs? Is training available at times to suit staff on a regular basis to ensure that maintenance of skills is ongoing?

In Andrew's case, there are a number of key aspects that are important for practitioners. It is vital to be aware of the key issues and challenges of your client group. However, as SLT your priority is to your clients and their communication needs. This means close liaison and collaboration with significant others in clients' lives as well as clients themselves. In addition, multidisciplinary goal setting and discussion can minimise risk. A good team should have a clear risk policy, where dealing with disclosures is discussed within a team framework, ensuring that clients are listened to. It appears that this situation has been dealt with too late, and it looks as if Andrew is going to have to engage in some serious discussion with Bill about his role and the requirements of his post, his actual level of competence, and his performance within the multidisciplinary team.

Celia Harding, Lecturer, Department of Language and Communication Science, City University London, UK

Commentary on Scenario 4.2

Judy Duchan

Things are not going well for any of the people in this scenario. The care worker (unnamed), speech-language pathologist (Andrew) and resident (Kieran) would probably agree that serious problems exist. Each, however, is likely to have a different take on what those problems are and what needs to be done to solve them.

⬜ The care worker would probably highlight low wages and/or lack of training to take care of the issues that come up, such as the one that Andrew is raising about the sexual activities of Kieran. Besides, there is no time nor is it their job to take care of such matters. Kieran is difficult enough to take care of, without having to deal with him about this touchy subject.

⬜ Andrew is likely to focus on his worries about Kieran's sexual activity. He fears that Kieran, his agency, and Kieran's possible sexual partner might be at risk for trouble or already in trouble. He feels something needs to be done immediately, but he doesn't know who should do it or what should be done. His efforts to talk to his team leader and the care worker have come to dead ends.

⬜ Kieran is obviously frustrated with his isolation and with the lack of responsiveness of his care workers. He feels like he is in jail – unable to communicate with anyone except Andrew and unable to get out, except for an occasional trip to the store or to town. He wants freedom and companionship, especially female companionship, and spends lots of time thinking about sex. He hopes Andrew will help him figure out a way he can meet a girl and spend some time with her.

The situation contains a number of serious problems that all need addressing. But what is the 'ethical dilemma' of the scenario? We can safely assume from the scenario that it is Kieran and his sexual activity that we are meant to focus on. Kieran's ambiguous message about sex is the most acute problem in the scenario. The other problems, such as low salary, insufficient time and unclear responsibilities, are more chronic. In the words of the scenario, it is the message from Kieran that gets the 'lights ... flashing in the Risk Assessment Section in Andrew's brain'.

So the acute ethical dilemma is what to do about Kiernan's ambiguous message. The solution to the dilemma, however, requires that we not see the situation as just about sex, but examine the chronic conditions that led to this particular acute problem. There are two that are apparent when reading between the lines of the scenario.

The first is that the staff and Kieran are not working together as a team and with Kieran to support him in his everyday activities and help him to lead an interesting, active life. This absence of team effort has led to the assumption that responsibility for the ethical dilemma should be assigned to a particular person. This assumption is expressed by Andrew when he asks for his team leader's help and also by the care worker, who says that the problem is neither hers nor Andrew's but belongs to the social worker.

My suggestion, then, would be that the staff find a way to meet regularly to create policies and procedures for how to handle issues such as these. This team could examine the policies and procedures of other agencies, such as those involved in mandated reporting about abuse, and fit them to their own specific needs. (See, e.g., Duchan, Calculator, Sonnenmeier, Diehl & Cumley, (2001), for a set of cautionary procedures that can be used when instituting controversial practices).

I suggest also that a support group for Kieran be formed, one similar to those involved in Personal Futures Planning programs (Mount, 1992; Mount & Zwernik, 1988). Such a group could offer Kieran opportunities to talk about his problems and hopes with people he can communicate with, people he trusts, people who care about him. This group could work with Kieran to help him to improve his current situation and achieve a better quality of life.

A second major problem evidenced in the scenario is that the members of the staff seem to regard Kieran as someone who is incompetent, irresponsible and in need of strict supervision to keep him out of trouble. These attitudes lead them to restrict Kieran's opportunities and to violate his basic rights: his right to be involved in his own decision making, his right to complain about his care, and his right to privacy. Such attitudes also result in the staff's failure to learn about and respond to Kieran's legitimate needs and requests. It might only be after Kieran became potentially dangerous to others or explosive that the staff would be forced to pay attention to him.

My recommendation is that the staff be trained to think of Kieran as a competent and worthy person with rights. This training could involve an outside agency, such as that provided in the Beyond Access Intervention (Jorgensen, McSheehan & Sonnenmeier, 2007), which works with groups to design support strategies based on a competence view of disability. The mantra of Beyond Access Intervention is the title of Ann Donnellan's (1984) paper 'The Criterion of the Least Dangerous Assumption', which presumes a positive view of a person, ascribing to him or her competence and goodwill and normal motives. In the case of Kieran, the training would also require staff to develop skills in communicating with someone with complex communication needs – including learning sign language.

The recommendations above (creating teams, support groups and training) all require a long-term effort and commitment from the staff and the organization. What, meanwhile, should be done to respond to the immediate ethical dilemma presented in the scenario, i.e. Kieran's ambiguous message and sexual needs?

In order to decide how to handle what may have happened, the ambiguous message needs disambiguation and corroboration. Andrew should go back to Kieran and talk again about what happened, trying to disambiguate the message. Andrew should then ask Kieran if he would be willing to talk with others about his sexual experience, preferably someone Kieran knows and trusts and can communicate with. If it turns out that Kieran has had or is having sexual relations with someone, the incident should be documented and reported and dealt with in terms of its particulars (whether the partner was consenting, whether they used protection, whether to provide sex education to Kieran, whether to allow it to continue). It should be dealt with sensitively, respectfully and in accordance with the legal guidelines of mandated reporting, if they exist.

I also recommend that the team leader, Bill, call his team together immediately, including the social worker, the care worker and Andrew, to talk about ways to support Kieran's communication and ways to expand his social opportunities. They should also involve Kieran in these discussions, whenever possible.

Judy Duchan, Professor Emeritus, State University of New York at Buffalo, USA

Discussion

At various points in this book we have discussed ethics in terms of being about more than 'A versus B' dilemmas. Factors such as subtlety of language, consideration of multiple participants and context-dependent interpretations of the 'truth' all serve to make ethics in healthcare much more multifaceted than the word 'dilemma' would suggest. In this chapter, however, we have a clear, though highly complex, example of a dilemma for the parents of Poppy as they consider whether to agree to cochlear implantation. Poppy either undergoes surgery or she doesn't. We discuss this issue first, before considering issues raised by long-term engagement with clients, ethical issues in teamwork, communication access and the therapist's role as 'Keeper of the Sign Store' and provider of helpful information.

Cochlear implantation

Scenario 4.1 illustrates the complex and emotional environment in which families must make decisions about intervention for their children with hearing impairment. As Fordham notes in her commentary, the majority of deaf children are born to hearing parents who want to communicate effectively with their deaf child and who worry about how the child will function in a hearing world. Poppy has the right to the best communication it is possible to achieve to enable her to function in the world. She also has a right to a life in which her sense of identity and community is robust.

Peter and Susan seem to have been presented by the CI centre and the Deaf community with an either/or choice: cochlear implantation or signing.

Before we go any further in this discussion, we should note the convention of using a capital letter to refer to the Deaf community, or the Deaf World as it is termed by some authors (Lane & Bahan, 1998). The capitalisation is also used to differentiate between those who use predominantly visual means of communication (given the opportunity) and people who are more readily described as hearing-impaired and who communicate primarily in spoken language. People in this latter group are unlikely to identify with the Deaf World, though of course there will be a range of views. The arguments presented below arise primarily from Deaf culture but serve to illustrate the deep ethical tensions surrounding CI technology.

The choice for Poppy's parents sits at the fulcrum between two strongly held ethical positions. Hearing people generally take the view that hearing is a normal state of affairs and that any limitation of it should be rectified if at all possible. Therefore, as discussed by Lane and Grodin (1997), the suggestion that intervention should be withheld – deliberately, so that a child can function as a member of the Deaf community – is deeply counterintuitive for hearing people. From the Deaf perspective, 'the single most recurrent criticism is that the surgery is unethical' (Lane & Grodin, 1997, p. 235), for precisely the same reasons, i.e. that it will remove Poppy from her culture (and in fact jeopardise the culture itself). As Christiansen and Leigh (2002) comment, ethical principles can be invoked to support either side of this argument.

For Poppy's parents, the perspective of the Deaf community has been brought home to them by the unsettling interactions with the deaf family at their church. The essence of their argument would be that surgery will remove both the imperative and the possibility for Poppy to learn to sign; she will therefore be cut off from her natural community and her future identity as a Deaf person. Although it is clearly not the *intent* of CI surgery to eradicate minority Deaf culture, the more successful the technique is, the more likely this becomes. The recognition and protection (in theory at least) given at national and international government levels to minority cultures and languages highlight this conflict of values even more starkly. Lane and Grodin (1997) provide a useful insight into this problem by identifying similarities with the ethical complexities of interracial adoption and *its* effect on minority cultures.

Important as the cultural implications of cochlear implantation are, the use of such technology also touches on the larger issue, which will undoubtedly increase in significance in the future, that of implant ethics in general. According to Hansson (2005), implant ethics refers to 'the study of ethical aspects of the lasting introduction of technological devices into the human body' (p. 519). It covers not only restoration of lost function (as in heart valve replacement) or absent function (such as with CI), but also the futuristic notion of capability enhancements, e.g. for military use. Central to debate on this subject is the fact that 'implant ethics . . . has to deal with issues of normality and disease, and with the admissibility of human enhancement' (Hansson, 2005, p. 521). To return to cochlear implantation, this raises the question of whether hearing impairment is indeed an impairment at all or is more akin to species variation in much the same way that skin colour is. This is a deeply political question; as Lane and Bahan (1998) assert, 'the political agenda of the Deaf World . . . more closely resembles the agenda of other language minorities than it does the agenda of any group of persons with a disability' (p. 298). A further interconnected controversy is the extent to which it is the role of healthcare to enhance and improve human functioning in any way possible, as opposed to treating and preventing problems/diseases/impairments. The Danish Deaf Association, for example, has expressed the opinion that deaf children are neither sick nor weak but happen to use a different language (in Nunes, 2001). Nunes also presents the other side of the debate, highlighting the fact that it might be seen as neglect or child abuse *not* to implant. Hansson (2005) comes down strongly on the latter side:

> *On balance, the Deaf World argument against cochlear implants is incompatible with well established principles of medical ethics. Physicians' responsibility towards individual*

patients cannot be defeated by the claims of a subculture that needs to recruit new members.
(p. 524)

These wider issues may be of no interest at all to Anthea and Peter as they contemplate their daughter's future. There are various other complicating factors, however, that also make this more than 'just' a fundamental clash of values. CI surgery does not by any means provide universally perfect hearing. As Van Dort notes in her commentary, the surgical process of cochlear implantation damages any residual hearing, removing the possibility of different intervention should technology improve in Poppy's lifetime. The risks of the surgery itself and of the possibility of subsequent failure of the CI need to be considered. The psychosocial concerns for families regarding surgery to the head also need to be understood, a point made by Fordham in her commentary. Just as with the ethics of interracial adoption, a balance has to be found between the rights of the individual child and those of the culture as a whole. Most implants are carried out for children of hearing parents, who are at a distance from Deaf culture. Levy (2002) argues that 'the significant disadvantages suffered by the hearing impaired can only be corrected by measures that would end Deaf culture' (p. 134), and that since the hearing parents of most potential implant recipients owe nothing to Deaf culture, society cannot ask them to forgo what they see as in the best interests of their children.

There is some hope that a convergence of positions can emerge. The stark choice of implantation or signing seems to be moderating, with an increasing trend towards integrated education, such that children receive intervention from both cochlear implantation and signing (Christiansen & Leigh, 2004) even in traditional bastions of signing and Deaf culture such as the Laurent Clerc National Deaf Education Centre within Gallaudet University in the USA. In the UK, research is under way into identification of good practice and the benefits of bilingual sign educational settings for children with CIs (Swanwick & Tsverik, 2007). If the CI centre in Scenario 4.1 can provide the evidence-based practice and flexibility that families deserve, implantation and signing may both be options for Poppy and her family. However, research seems increasingly to support the finding that best results in speech and language acquisition are achieved with implantation before 24 months of age (Nicholas & Geers, 2007). Thus, although the starkness of the choice for Peter and Anthea may be moderated by the possibility of essentially bilingual approaches, they still need to make a decision soon about implantation for Poppy.

Spare a thought at this point for Susan, faced with Anthea's direct question. What would Susan do if Poppy were *her* daughter? Susan somehow has to demonstrate recognition of the intent of the question (an appeal for help), convey empathy and understanding, empower the parents in their difficult decision making, and provide information in a manner the parents can grasp. Simultaneously she must avoid conveying any of her own biases or reservations about the intervention being considered or the impact the parents' decision may have on her own practice. She also has to negotiate the subtleties of answering or not answering the direct question. There are clear reasons not to answer the question, not least because a direct response serves to transfer some of the responsibility for the decision to Susan, an uncomfortable position if things do not turn out as hoped. In addition, Anthea may allow her trust in Susan to outweigh other evidence. For Anthea, though, this is a straightforward question from one human being to another, and the apparent veil of professionalism preventing a straightforward answer may seem particularly ethically flimsy from where she is sitting. Susan must weigh up all these factors and respond appropriately within a few seconds.

Long-term engagement

The difficulty for Susan in responding to Anthea's direct question is compounded by the established nature of their relationship. Susan knows Poppy's family from a previous therapeutic relationship with Poppy's brother, and, as is often the case in country towns, Susan and Poppy's mother Anthea have another (albeit limited) dimension to their relationship, as mothers of preschool children. Likewise, in the second scenario, Andrew has been working with Kieran for some time. As a result he knows Kieran's preferred topics of communication, interprets his signs fairly well, and has built up rapport and trust with him.

SLTs working in the disability sector, in contrast to those (including SLTs) working in acute medical settings, tend to have prolonged engagement with clients and their families. Long-term relationships are beneficial for clients and professionals in many ways. They can enable professionals to have a more holistic view of the client, more able to see them as part of a larger context (Bronfenbrenner, 1994). This can help the therapist to make better decisions about management and to present options in ways more likely to be understood and accepted by families. Satisfaction of families with services and of professionals in interaction with families and clients can be higher as a result (Dunst, Trivette & Deal, 1994).

However, these levels of familiarity and comfort can also be problematic. Anthea may understandably have higher expectations of a straight response to her direct question because of her established relationship with Susan. High levels of familiarity may allow over-identification or a sense of 'knowing what's best for this family' to creep in to the professional's thinking. Familiarity may also blind professionals to the boundaries of their role (Egan, 1990) and to changes in needs or attitudes of clients, family members or other staff. While empathy and care are important aspects of healthcare practice, they should not override professionals' key role to support families to make their own decisions (Dunst et al., 1994). Harding suggests that in Scenario 4.2 Andrew may have disengaged from the carers and resigned himself to a belief that the care staff will not extend themselves on Kieran's behalf. Andrew may also have overstepped the boundaries of his role as SLT in Kieran's residence. He has perhaps come to believe that he knows what is best for Kieran and has not recognised that Kieran's needs for more freedom, autonomy and privacy need to be managed in a collaborative way with others.

Teamwork

It is very difficult in modern healthcare for individual members of staff to work in complete isolation, and staff in general are exhorted to work in teams for the benefit of patients. Indeed, 'the value of teamwork is taken for granted by health care professionals' (Cott, 1998, p. 848). Positive as this expected level of teamwork may potentially be, it is a long way from exhortation to effective functioning in the long term. Given the complex dynamics of even the smallest teams, teamwork in all areas of healthcare is fertile ground for ethical complexity. Both commentators on Scenario 4.2 identify the fact that issues raised by Kieran's possible sexual activity are likely to be only a surface manifestation of deeper problems, in that 'the staff and Kieran are not working together as a team' (Duchan).

Opie (1997) presents a depressingly long list of potential problems encountered in teamwork, a small selection of which includes inadequate organisational support, lack of continuity of members, difficulty in defining key terms and lack of interprofessional trust. Perhaps the most important item on the list, though, is a lack of clear goals. When clinicians and administration staff who managed admissions to an acute rehabilitation hospital were surveyed about ethical concerns in their workplace, team conflict around goal setting was identified as the second most common ethical problem (Kirschner, Stocking, Wagner, Foye & Siegler., 2001) (the first, in a private healthcare system, being reimbursement). Lack of clear goal setting may be evident at any level from day-to-day working with individual clients to the deepest levels of team purpose. Thus it is quite possible that the apparent difficulty of the team in Scenario 4.2 in agreeing how to work with Kieran reflects a deeper difficulty in agreeing why the team exists in the first place, or, indeed, a complete lack of discussion of why the team exists. A fundamental issue here is that any group of people working in close proximity can assume or be presented with the label of 'team' without consideration of what that means. In essence, unless the group of people have explicitly identified shared goals at multiple levels, and shared understandings of what each member of the team should (or may) contribute to those goals, then their existence as a team is precarious. In fact it is often illuminating, particularly in terms of gaps in service delivery for individual clients, to ask team members what they think the other members' roles are. The chances of shared ethical agendas, a common direction and shared responses to problems are inevitably compromised unless these discussions are had at the time the team is formed, are discussed with new members, are regularly revised and are open to scrutiny and challenge. It seems likely that Kieran's team has not discussed his sexual needs and rights, much less decided who should take what role.

Cott (1998), examining team structures in a long-term residential care facility, identified two starkly different ways of working for care staff and 'multidisciplinary professional' staff. The former she described as having 'simple role-sets, minimal involvement in team decision-making and ritualistic orientations towards their work and teamwork'; the latter, on the other hand, had 'complex role-sets, greater involvement in team decision-making and organic orientations towards their work and teamwork (p. 848). Whether any of the characters in Scenario 4.2 is working to these agendas is unknown, but Cott's description suggests that the teams she studied will also experience organisational and ethical challenges.

Kieran's team does not seem able to emphasise holistic models of care for its client, an important goal for healthcare teams (Boon, Verhoef, O'Hara & Findlay, 2004). Further, a key indicator of successful residential care programmes (Mansell, 2006) – staff support for residents to engage in meaningful activity – is low in this team. As Team Leader, Bill has ethical obligations to facilitate more effective functioning by his team members, both for their own professional and personal development and ultimately for the benefit of residents like Kieran. This is not an easy call for Bill, and as Epstein-Frish, van Dam and Chenoweth (2006, #257, p. 11) note in their discussion of the evidence base for best practice in accommodation and support for people with disability, staff in supervisory positions in residential care need to be given training, support and supervision to:

- lead direct staff in positive behaviour support and technical aspects of support for people with disability;
- implement methods for staff: resident deployment and activity planning;
- and monitor quality of support provided to people with disability.

Access to communication

In Scenario 4.2 the lack of clarity in the client's signed communications and lack of communication skill on the part of his carers contribute to the ethical difficulty. While sign systems of deaf communities around the world are rich and sophisticated, and allow for complex and nuanced communications, sign systems such as Makaton (Grove & Walker, 1990) for people with intellectual impairments are often necessarily taught at a basic level and often used in unsophisticated ways. Sign language is vulnerable to misinterpretation if placement, handshaping and plane of movement are not accurate (Conlin, Mirus, Mauk & Meier, 2000). Moreover, readers themselves must have an extensive sign repertoire, must be able to recognise any idiosyncratic forms of the signs made by different users and must be aware of the range of possible topics and meanings their interlocutor may be interested in communicating about. This is the technical problem with which Andrew finds himself. He is a proficient signer and appears to know Kieran well enough to recognise and interpret his signs; he is also well aware that sex is one of Kieran's favourite topics. But even so, the ambiguity of sign language or the proficiency with which Kieran selects and shapes his signs, or in all likelihood both factors, have created lack of clarity in the communication. As a consequence, there is lack of clarity on how to proceed in managing the multiple ethical issues involved.

There is an additional ethical element to Andrew's communication with Kieran. As the SLT, Andrew may well have control of the choice of signs to teach Kieran and his carers. He is in essence the 'Keeper of the Sign Store'. He can ration out signs and censor topics as he sees fit, for example by not teaching Kieran signs related to sexual activity or swearing. The ethical undertones of teaching sign language are not well considered in speech and language therapy literature, though there are some discussions in the literature of related fields such as education (B. Jones, Clark & Stolz, 1997), professional sign language interpreting (Tate & Turner, 1997) and sign language interpreting with vulnerable populations such as in mental health services for people with hearing loss (Gutman, 2005). Metzger (1999), for example, suggests that neutrality in sign language interpreting is a myth. This literature could serve to alert SLTs to their power and responsibility in clinical practice. Our decisions about what we see as appropriate signs (and therefore topics of communication) for our clients may unwittingly restrict adult clients' rights to participate in normal adult activities and interests.

Provision of information

Earlier in this section we touched on the factors that Susan needs to balance in constructing her response to Anthea, mother of Poppy. Susan also needs to consider the wider implications of provision of information to clients and families to facilitate their autonomous decision making about how to proceed with intervention or planning for the future.

In Scenario 4.1, Poppy's parents need information to help them make a difficult decision. Although at one level this requires exchange of information, it is only necessary to consider the influence of, say, tone of voice on the recipient of a potentially negative diagnosis to recognise the ethical dimensions of providing vulnerable people with information. To quote from a poem by Jenny Lewis (2002), one of a series about her breast cancer, 'All that technical data so patiently explained, falls before us in a sombre harvest to be winnowed blindly for the magic words' (p. 166). The information provided for Anthea and Peter need not necessarily be sombre but it is certainly serious.

Christiansen and Leigh (2002) suggest that for parents to make informed choices about cochlear implantation they need comprehensive information, an awareness of the value judgements of the people providing the information, and an understanding of how those people ultimately interpret the information they are providing. Aspects of informational counselling – how, when and in what format they receive information from people holding different perspectives – will be of central importance for Peter and Anthea. As discussed in Chapter 2, Seedhouse (1998, 2001, 2002b) views access to meaningful information as one of the key requirements for health.

Much of the research into information counselling has come from genetic counselling and counselling for patients with cancer. However, there is an emerging body of literature from or directly pertinent to speech and language therapy. Provision of information has been found to reduce carer stress in head injury (Blake, 2008; Morris, 2001) and in aphasia (Brumfitt, Atkinson & Greated, 1994; Wiles, Pain, Buckland & McLellan, 1998). Writing on the role of nurses in information counselling for families of people experiencing stroke, van der Smagt-Duijnstee, Hamers, Abu-Saad and Zuidhof (2001) report relatives' statements that their most important need was for questions to be answered honestly. However, as we note in Chapter 5, it can be difficult to provide accurate information about the future when that future is some way off and unclear. Information may need to be delivered in a staged manner in accord with progress of the patient. The timing of information counselling is critical. Provided too early, it may raise anxiety unnecessarily or be partially or completely forgotten in the midst of a crisis state, such as when confronting serious illness or injury or making a crucial decision for one's child. Provided too late, it may be received after events have been set in train without patients or parents understanding or contributing.

The format in which information is provided is also important for health professionals to consider. Research into informational counselling for women with breast cancer suggests that videotaped information followed by opportunities for discussion is an effective way of delivering information to women about surgical options and of addressing misunderstandings and distress which arise from viewing the videotape (Cull et al., 1998), and that consultants still must take care to address patients' emotional as well as informational needs (Lobb et al., 2004). Professionals need to monitor carefully clients' readiness for, understanding of and acceptance of information if they are to truly empower them.

Summary

This chapter has highlighted several ethical issues that may arise in speech and language therapy practice beyond those inherent in direct interactions with clients. SLTs and other staff are often in a position to function as mediators and facilitators of communication for clients with intellectual and sensory impairments; in the process their actions can facilitate access to normal communication opportunities as part of a fulfilling life, or they can serve to restrict those same communication opportunities. Scenario 4.2 featuring Susan and Anthea also highlights the power of subtle uses of communication with clients.

The value and risks of long-term engagement with clients and their families have also been considered in this chapter. Prolonged engagement can facilitate more holistic perspectives on clients' and families' needs but may also lead to complacency or inertia in perceiving changing needs and perspectives.

Speech and language therapy with people who have intellectual and sensory impairments is characterised by the complexities of working in teams. Taking teamwork practice for granted can exacerbate the risk of ethical difficulties in team settings.

5 Acquired communication disorders

Introduction

The term 'acquired communication disorders' – the focus of this chapter – could conceivably cover any disorder of communication not present from birth, so some initial narrowing of focus is warranted. Generally speaking, the term is applied to (a) communication disorders arising in adolescence or adulthood (though see Lees, 2005, for discussion of, e.g., aphasia in children) and (b) communication disorders of neurogenic origin, thereby excluding fields such as voice disorder. The two groups of people we highlight here are those with aphasia and those who have communication disorders as a result of traumatic brain injury (TBI). Acquired communication disorders that arise from degenerative conditions are discussed in Chapter 7.

Recent figures from the American Speech-Language-Hearing Association (ASHA, 2008d) give an overall sense of the numbers of people with aphasia. The report estimates that in the USA 80,000 people acquire aphasia per year, resulting in approximately one million people living with the condition. This prevalence rate (in a population of just over 300 million) is equivalent to about 0.3% of the population and it does not seem unreasonable to extrapolate this percentage to other countries (e.g. 200,000 people with aphasia in the UK). An alternative way of looking at this is that in the USA this is equivalent (very approximately) to 10 people with aphasia for every single qualified SLT in the country (ASHA, 2007). We leave readers to do the rest of the arithmetic relating to all those therapists who do not work in aphasia and for countries with much lower ratios of SLTs to population.

Achieving meaningful estimates of numbers of people with communication disorder arising from TBI is more difficult since the underlying concepts and even terminology are still subject to debate. Body and Perkins (2006) highlight the varied terms (cognitive-linguistic, complex, high-level) in use to describe communication after TBI, and the difficulty of defining what constitutes a communication disorder is illustrated by the absence of established standardised assessments (Turkstra, Coelho & Ylvisaker, 2005).

It is undoubtedly the case that the number of people sustaining TBI is very high in many countries. For example, in the USA it has been estimated that 1.4 million people sustain a TBI each year and 5.3 million Americans live with its effects (Centers for Disease Control, 2008). It is also well established that disruption of cognition (in particular, attention, memory and the executive functions) is almost unavoidable to some degree. The intricate relationship between cognition and communication in TBI has been recognised since the 1980s (Hagen, 1982; Prigatano, Roueche & Fordyce, 1985), as has the widespread social isolation experienced by people after such injury. The causal chain, with communication as a central link, is fairly clear.

Major changes have occurred in aphasia therapy and the SLT's role over the last decade or so (though developments have been taken up differently across the world). One change has been the development of the cognitive neuropsychological model as a possible basis for assessment and intervention (Byng, Kay, Edmundson & Scott, 1990). Another perhaps even more significant shift has been a new focus on the social implications of aphasia and on efforts to support people with aphasia both to participate in social activity to a greater extent and, crucially, to contribute to the development of these and other aphasia services (Cruice, 2007; Pound, Duchan, Penman, Hewitt & Parr, 2007).

SLT involvement in intervention after TBI has long been a multidisciplinary affair, requiring complex cross-party discussion and negotiation. Techniques from other disciplines, most notably clinical (neuro)psychology, have been incorporated into the work of SLTs (Ylvisaker & Feeney, 1998). As with aphasia therapy, focus has widened to include conversational partners and the wider community, for example training police personnel in the management of interactions with brain-injured people (Togher, McDonald, Code & Grant, 2004). One significant aspect of rehabilitation after TBI, applying to speech and language therapy and other disciplines alike, is exemplified by the self-explanatory *Whatever It Takes* model described by Willer and Corrigan (1994).

Stroke and TBI share the key characteristic of sudden, unexpected and usually dramatic onset. The accompanying sudden suspension of cognitive and/or communicative ability (not to mention physical sequelae) necessitates equally sudden transfer of responsibilities to other people, whether acute medical staff or relatives and friends. The balance between re-establishment of personal control and the responsibilities that are held by other people is a feature of both the scenarios in this chapter.

Scenario 5.1

The first scenario in this chapter is based on Julianna, who has been receiving therapy for aphasia following a stroke and who has now been placed on review by her therapist. Julianna's husband has decided to take up the issue in the form of a letter.

11 Birch Close
Middleton

Miss M. Sharma
Specialist Speech Therapist

Dear Miss Sharma

I am writing on behalf of my wife, for whom – as you know – the challenge of constructing such a letter would currently be very significant, a marked contrast to her previous achievements in the field of commerce. In addition, Julianna fell in the garden last week and has strapping on her wrist.

At the speech therapy appointment on 17 May we were both somewhat taken aback to be informed that no further service would be available until a review appointment in September. I appreciate the fact that you took the trouble to speak to me after the session with Julianna. Having returned home and reflected on the situation I have reached the conclusion that the decision to suspend therapy after ten sessions is (a) entirely unsatisfactory and (b) founded on unsubstantial evidence, or possibly no evidence at all. I have worked in healthcare for long enough to know that major progress has been made in basing provision on sound evidence and I see no reason why speech therapy should not be subject to the same demands.

My wife enjoyed her sessions with you and I have noted a number of improvements which I think are a direct result of her attendance. For example, having previously been unable to name our grandchildren, she surprised everyone at a recent family gathering by saying both their names spontaneously. This gave the entire occasion a considerable boost. I am sure you realise how important such seemingly small gains can be. More importantly, she has applied herself to the 'homework' you gave her with a degree of energy she has been unable to summon for any other activity since the stroke.

Despite these gains, Julianna remains severely restricted in her communication ability. She is unable to discuss anything complicated, to deal with anyone coming to the door, to write a shopping list, to follow a recipe or to talk on the telephone to our son working in Kuwait. In addition she remains very emotional and cries at the slightest provocation, even when I endeavour to assist her with her communication exercises. Since I am unable to leave the house without Julianna, I have had to suspend all activities other than caring for her. I am unsure how the speech and language therapy service perceives this level of communication to be tolerable and thus compatible with the suspension of therapy.

You made the suggestion that Julianna should perhaps consider joining the Stroke Group described in your leaflet. I do not think it would be either appropriate or helpful for her to meet with people she does not know in order to have a conversation, particularly since this is exactly the activity she finds hardest. Furthermore, if it is conversation that my wife needs, I am perfectly capable of conducting one with her myself.

As noted above, my complaint is not about your therapy; rather it is about the impending absence of it. I would be grateful if you could discuss this issue with your manager at the earliest opportunity. Should it prove impossible for the speech and language therapy service to reconsider the decision to terminate therapy, I wonder if you would be amenable to the idea of visiting my wife on a private basis at a time to suit you.

Yours sincerely

Dr J. Jankowski
cc Clive Marner, Manager, Speech and Language Therapy
   Louise Chan, Chief Executive, Middleton & Duffield Healthcare

Commentary on Scenario 5.1

Leanne Togher

Terminating treatment for people with aphasia has become an increasingly vexing and problematic issue for speech pathologists around the world, particularly given the diminishing healthcare budget for chronic conditions. Indeed, it has been suggested that some people with aphasia should never be discharged, given the profound impact that this disability can have on everyday life. This letter raises a number of issues.

Advocacy for people with aphasia

Julianna is lucky that she has an intelligent advocate who can write a letter of complaint about her discontinuation of treatment. It raises concerns, however, for those who do not have an advocate and therefore have no redress when their treatment is suspended. While self-help and advocacy groups are continuing to emerge (such as the Australian Aphasia Association), people with aphasia still rely on having internet access or contact with someone to connect them with these groups. Although the clinician had referred Julianna to a stroke group, this was not what she and her husband wanted. Rather, they were looking for ongoing intervention for her communication. The problem here is a lack of availability of clinical services for people with aphasia in the medium to long term. This has led to another avenue pursued by some clinicians, to create longer-term services with the help of volunteers. This can be effective, but it is a major enterprise to set up and sustain. Finally, aphasia research clinics and long-term group programs can also fill the gap left by a lack of services.

Service delivery model

The suspension of treatment was a surprise to Julianna and her husband, suggesting that there was little communication regarding the treatment plan or the discharge process. Perhaps Ms Sharma wanted to wait and see how Julianna progressed in treatment before deciding on a course of action. However, it appears that there was a 10-week course of treatment followed by a three-month break, and that this was determined before the first session had started. Certainly, it raises the issue that the manner of provision of speech pathology services and the discharge process should be discussed at the beginning of the treatment program. With the knowledge that there are only 10 weeks on offer followed by a three-month break, there are clear implications regarding goal setting, particularly when taking the person's communication needs into account.

Decision to discharge

Dr Jankowski raises the issue of the evidence used to suspend treatment. There are increasing reports suggesting that treatment for people with chronic aphasia can be effective. The decision to discharge did not appear to be based on observations that Julianna was functionally able to participate in everyday life, as she still presents with profound social disability as a result of her aphasia. As the evidence base for speech pathology treatments increases, it will be increasingly demonstrated that 'no treatment' can lead to negative consequences, in contrast to treatments that improve quality of life (Robey, 1994). It is therefore not inconceivable that health authorities could face legal action in cases where the best treatment was not applied.

Measurement of progress

This case raises the issue that the way treatment progress is measured may influence the decision to discharge. Julianna's husband indicates that being able to name the grandchildren is a significant and important gain. However, this functional progress may not have translated into improved scores on standardized assessment protocols and this may have contributed to the three-month suspension of treatment. Dr Jankowski refers to the ability to say the grandchildren's names spontaneously as 'seemingly small gains', possibly reflecting the way the clinician had referred to them. This raises the issue that clinicians must be keenly aware of what the valued communication contexts are for people with aphasia, and, particularly, the interpersonal roles they want to assume outside the treatment room. In Julianna's case, this is likely to be grandmother, wife and mother, as well as active member of the community, assuming she is unable to return to her previous work. Dealing with scenarios such as answering the front door, writing a shopping list and following a recipe may all have been achievable. If goals had been set up differently at the beginning of treatment, the achievement of saying the grandchildren's names spontaneously might have been viewed as a major milestone rather than a small gain.

Emotional support for Julianna

It is unclear whether Julianna is depressed or labile, but this raises the issue of access to other support such as counselling. It appears that after the last session all contact with the health service was going to cease until September. It might be appropriate at this stage for Julianna to be referred for some form of ongoing emotional support, even in the absence of ongoing speech therapy. The dilemma here is that it will be difficult for Julianna to express her feelings and thoughts, but nonetheless, a counsellor who is trained in using alternative and augmentative communication could contribute significantly to Julianna's ability to adjust to her communication disability.

Additional support for Julianna's husband

It appears that there is no support for Dr Jankowski as the primary carer for his wife, either from a practical or from an emotional perspective. Resources are limited for carers, but Dr Jankowski may be in the position to pay for some respite to enable him to engage in other activities.

Nature of the homework

It is concerning that Dr Jankowski refers to 'homework' in inverted commas. It implies that this resembled school work, and possibly did not include communication partner training, but rather focused on the language impairment. Given Dr Jankowski's willingness to converse with his wife, it might have been of greater use to focus some of the treatment on him rather than his wife. That is, time spent training him, using a program such as *Supporting Partners of People with Aphasia in Relationships and Conversation* (Lock & Wilkinson, 2001), might have been of more benefit than focusing all treatment tasks on Julianna.

Treating people as private cases while working in a public health system

A conflict of interest is introduced for Ms Sharma if she pursues this avenue. For example, when September comes around, does she discontinue seeing Julianna as a private case? Would it be tempting for her simply to continue seeing Julianna privately rather than reviewing her in the public system? This final issue is difficult and poses an ethical dilemma for clinicians, particularly those who work part-time in both public and private sectors. In Sydney, public health clinicians see people privately only if they live in a different health sector to the one in which they work. However, the issue becomes more difficult for those who live and work in a large rural or remote health region. At the very least, it is critical that the ability to pay privately does not deprive the person of public health resources.

Provision of long-term services to people with chronic aphasia has led to the development of several novel initiatives; however, these are typically available in large cities and require additional resources, time and energy that may not be available to clinicians like Ms Sharma. Nonetheless, the advent of partner training programs and the acknowledgment that people with aphasia can respond to treatment in the chronic phase suggest that speech pathologists have an obligation to seek out ways to provide long-term communication options for this population.

Leanne Togher, Senior Research Fellow, National Health and Medical Research Council, Faculty of Health Sciences, The University of Sydney, Australia

Commentary on Scenario 5.1

Madeline Cruice

This scenario describes a husband's discontent with the apparent abrupt end of speech and language therapy treatment for his wife, for which they were unprepared. The cessation of therapy appears unfounded and unreasonable to the husband given his wife's significant ongoing communication needs. While Julianna has been motivated, it suggests that she has made very little progress over the 10 sessions. We assume therapy has focused on improving her language function, with the husband observing the sessions. Julianna's significant everyday communication needs, as described by her husband, suggest that therapy has either intentionally not addressed these needs or that what she has been doing in therapy has had no impact on real life yet. There is a concern that the letter might reflect only the husband's wishes, as well as a concern that he may be overprotective or even controlling in making decisions about what could be helpful for his wife (e.g. the Stroke Group). It appears that Julianna is upset and may even be depressed by her communication difficulties, and is dependent on her husband now, which raises concerns about her individual safety in the home and community. The situation has significantly changed their lifestyles, with the husband caring full-time for his wife, presumably because of communication concerns. (Note that while the husband alludes to his wife's fall in the garden, his letter does not suggest that she has difficulty walking, going to the toilet or preparing meals, which would typically indicate full-time caring needs.) Finally, we assume no other allied health or social care professionals are involved in this case.

What are the issues and why do they present challenges?

The abrupt termination of treatment presents as a challenge because preparing clients and carers for discharge is part of our standard practice. The second issue is the apparent lack of evidence or explicit reasoning for terminating therapy. This presents as a challenge because a therapist is required to be accountable to the client and carer (as well as the healthcare manager) and to be able to justify the decisions made and the course of action taken. The third main issue is the termination of therapy without a sufficient review of the client's life situation and her current concerns and needs. This presents as a challenge because a therapist is required to consider what risks there may be of *not* providing therapy to a client, which necessitates undertaking a case review. It is clear that the therapist has not identified Julianna's significant functional communication disability or has chosen not to focus on it. Nor has the therapist identified Julianna's emotional state or her dependency on her husband. This is a concern because a therapist is required to address a client's emotional and psychological needs as well as the communication needs. It is especially important because emotional state is thought to influence progress in therapy. The above issues are particularly challenging since the therapist concerned is in a senior position, which we infer from her 'specialist' title, and thus more would be expected of her given her level of knowledge and skills (i.e. complying with best practice documents, current position papers and clinical guidelines). Finally, the husband's request for private speech therapy from the therapist herself raises a concern because of the pre-existing relationship between the therapist and client in public service provision, and because we assume that Julianna has been discharged on the basis of *no further improvement demonstrated in therapy*. Given this rationale for termination, it would thus be contradictory to agree to provide further speech therapy privately.

There are several reasons the abovementioned issues might have arisen. It seems that no explicit discussion of how therapy provision would be determined has taken place – that is, whether therapy is structured around clear goals and contingent on Julianna making sufficient progress towards these goals, and thus would be discontinued if she ceased to make progress; or contingent on what the Trust could provide, such as 10 weeks of therapy sessions only. Furthermore, it would seem that no therapy contract (with goals, time frame and monitoring checks) has been communicated to and shared with the client and carer. Nor has a discharge report been written, or if it has, it does not clearly communicate the reasons for terminating therapy. It is possible that the therapist was unable to justify continued therapy (targeting the goals that were initially chosen) if she had identified that Julianna was not making progress, but that she had not made her reasoning clear to client and carer. It is possible that the health provider had a role in terminating therapy. In light of the ongoing challenge of managing scarce resources in modern healthcare, changing demands on the therapist's (or team's) caseload or reductions in staffing might have meant that this client was no longer a priority. The scenario suggests that the therapy undertaken, while not dissatisfying to the carer, may not have been initially informed by client and carer's priorities. Furthermore, it implies that the therapist did not undertake a functional communication assessment or conduct a home visit prior to ending therapy to gather information about Julianna's life situation to inform the decision-making process. It seems that Julianna and her husband are not linked in to their GP, her hospital consultant or key worker, who might have identified their emotional and psychological needs. Finally, it is possible that the carer and client have not been able to take on board the information, advice, suggestions, and so on, given the crisis event of having a stroke and the process of learning to live with its consequences.

The following are some suggested actions that the therapist could have taken in managing Julianna's case. The therapist could have sought both Julianna's and her husband's perceptions of her communication difficulties and their priorities during the initial assessment process. There is also an increasing shift in clinical practice to involve clients in setting goals for therapy. It is recommended that therapists *discuss* with clients and *document* the nature, purpose and likely outcome of therapy using a goal-oriented approach. This could be used to track Julianna's progress regularly throughout therapy, and thus would facilitate ongoing discussion of her progress towards goals (or not) and ongoing identification of needs or modification of goals, preparing both Julianna and her husband adequately for discharge, transfer or onward referral to another service/agency. If the Trust does indeed limit provision, it is important to discuss this openly with the client and carer and to determine what is achievable in the time frame. We have assumed that therapy focused on language, but the therapist could have considered other intervention options, including functional therapy focusing on everyday communicative activities (such as following a recipe), teaching compensatory strategies such as maximising Julianna's skills in drawing and gesture, and working with her husband to maximise his skills as a communication partner. If service provision within the Trust is time-limited (e.g. 10 weeks only and not dependent on the client's ongoing need), it is appropriate to recommend private speech and language therapy, and the therapist should provide contact details for the Association of Speech and Language Therapists in Independent Practice or a similar private practice organisation. Finally, clients and family members often need support to appreciate the benefits of community stroke groups and to muster the confidence to try something new. One way of demonstrating (rather than discussing) this, and addressing client and carer's concerns, is to arrange to go to the Stroke Group together. This would entail mental and practical preparation before going, facilitating conversation on the day, and discussing the experience afterwards.

With hindsight we can reflect on what actions could have been taken. However, the information revealed in the husband's letter has implications for actions that need to be taken now. There are three main issues that the therapist is now aware of, and will need to address as part of her duty of care to this client given the risk that they pose for Julianna's and her husband's wellbeing. They are: (a) Julianna's significant communication disability affecting her safety when alone at home (among other important functional communication needs) as well as in the community; (b) her and her husband's emotional distress and need for support; and (c) a concern around her dependency and possible lack of autonomy to make decisions about activities in her life. Further speech and language therapy is implicated, with clear goals to improve Julianna's functional communication and safety so that she can gain more independence from her husband and improve her quality of life. Their emotional and psychological needs may be addressed in therapy or referral to another professional may be warranted.

Madeline Cruice, Senior Lecturer, Department of Language and Communication Science, City University London, UK

Scenario 5.2

We now shift our attention from aphasia to focus on traumatic brain injury. The scenario is presented in the form of a discharge report for Dean Taverner who has been on a hospital rehabilitation ward for the last couple of months following a road traffic accident.

Middleton Hospital: Ward 12
Discharge Report

Name: Dean Taverner   **Sex:** Male/Female

Date of Birth: 04.06.81   **Presenting Condition:** traumatic brain injury

Date of Admission: 25.06.08   **Date of Report:** 01.09.08

History of present condition

Dean was involved in a road traffic accident on 23.05.08 (age: 26) when the car he was driving left the road at a bend and hit a tree. No other vehicles were involved. The front seat passenger (Maria Bianchi = Dean's partner) died in the car. The back seat passenger (Paul Bianchi = Maria's brother) sustained minor cuts and bruises.

Dean was initially admitted to Blackton Hall Hospital, where his Glasgow Coma Scale score on arrival was recorded as 6/15. He was intubated and ventilated. CT scan showed 'extensive brain injury with bilateral fronto-parietal contusions and blood in the posterior horn of both lateral ventricles and around the brainstem region'. In addition to the brain injury, Dean suffered a left pneumothorax, fracture of the radius and ulna of the left arm and facial lacerations. He remained in coma until 17.06.08 (25 days) and was transferred to Ward 12 on 25.06.08 (33 days post-injury).

Note: Dean has been interviewed on two occasions by police in relation to the accident. Staff from Social Work and Psychology have been present at each interview. The police interviewers are aware that Dean's memory for events in the week prior to the injury is not consistently reliable.

Social background

Prior to injury Dean lived with Maria and their son Kyle, now aged four. Dean will be discharged to the care of his mother, Maureen Taverner. Mrs Taverner has a number of health issues and is currently not in paid employment. Staff in the Social Work Department are investigating sources of financial support for Dean and his mother as a matter of urgency.

Kyle is currently living with Maria Bianchi's parents. Dean has a strong attachment to Kyle and is committed to caring for him independently at some point in the future. It is known (by staff but not by Dean) that Mr and Mrs Bianchi may contest this on the basis of Dean's capacity to take responsibility for Kyle.

Note: Dean's mother has categorically refused to house Dean's tarantula, which is being cared for by a friend. This is a source of friction between Dean and Mrs Taverner.

At the time of injury Dean was working as a motor mechanic at J.C. Motors. He has no formal educational qualifications. His stated aim is to open his own garage and run it as an independent business. Dean's leisure interests include taking part in motocross and watching horse racing. Mrs Taverner has requested that staff working with Dean actively discourage him from placing bets.

General presentation

Dean is generally sociable and seeks out company. He has a lively sense of humour, though this is not always socially appropriate. Dean has a good relationship with his son, who has made weekly visits to the hospital in the company of Mrs Taverner.

Dean is easily distracted from activities and conversations. He is prone to significant verbal outbursts and has twice directed physical aggression at other patients on the ward. He expresses a firm opinion that he will be able to live independently with Kyle and run his own business. However, he also repeatedly seeks agreement from staff that both these plans will be successful and tends to become verbally aggressive if agreement is not forthcoming.

Speech and language therapy

Key Points:

- ▒ basic auditory comprehension and verbal expression abilities intact
- ▒ mild dysarthria characterised by reduced breath support for speech, reduced accuracy of articulation at speed and mild hypernasality
- ▒ socially inappropriate comments
- ▒ repetition of limited range of topics:
  - – taking legal action against the council for the state of the road surface
  - – cars he has driven/will drive
  - – working for himself (as opposed to 'being a wage slave')
  - – looking after Kyle

Input has covered three primary areas:

Motor speech: Therapy has been conducted in the gym during timetabled physiotherapy sessions, working on postural control, breath support and articulation. Dean is able to improve his breath support and articulation when fully focused on this as a task, sometimes when prompted during conversation (away from the gym) and when angry.

Socially inappropriate comments: Dean expresses a generally low (and sometimes offensive) opinion of women, including Maria. It has been strongly conveyed to Dean that the latter is not acceptable.

Dean has made sexual comments to and about female staff, though there has been no evidence of sexually disinhibited physical behaviour. Dean was initially unenthusiastic – and at times antagonistic – about attending speech and language therapy but has become more compliant in recent weeks. His willingness to attend therapy has been accompanied by an increase in sexually based jokes and references to the therapist's private life. A policy has been instigated with all staff of not responding to these remarks; this has resulted in a mild decrease in the behaviour over the last month.

Topic repetitiveness: Therapy has focused on encouraging a wider range of topics for Dean to initiate, in order to restrict his use of repeated topics. (It has become apparent that some of the other ward patients are beginning to avoid Dean.) Dean agrees in theory that it is preferable to have a variety of subjects to talk about but maintains that each car he has driven/will drive represents a different topic, in addition to which he sees an ability to discuss cars in detail as crucial to his future plans for owning a garage. Despite some progress in background discussion and in role play during therapy sessions, Dean sometimes starts up a favourite topic with whoever he meets on leaving therapy.

Dean has asked for assistance in keeping track of information in the racing papers in order to place more advantageous bets. To date it has been possible not to meet this request since ward routines have prevented Dean from being in a position to make bets easily. This situation is likely to become more problematic once Dean is in the community.

Note: During two speech and language therapy sessions Dean has disclosed that he and Paul Bianchi smoked marijuana immediately prior to the accident. However, he has denied this during interview with the police.

Commentary on Scenario 5.2

Leanne Togher

Traumatic brain injury is a catastrophic event that typically happens to young men like Dean with their life in front of them. Up until their accident they are in control of their circumstances, choosing who they live with, where they work, whether they have children and, if they have children, how to care for them. By the age of 26 most people have taken responsibility for their lives and are living independently. This also means they are responsible for their own failings and misdemeanours as well. The striking aspect of Dean's story is that all this comes to a complete halt with his accident. As well as sustaining a severe injury, he has lost his partner (and mother of his child), he has a changed relationship with his son, he is going to have to live with his mother, he is unable to work and, radically, he has changed from being an independent person to losing control over the most basic rights. It is little wonder that people with TBI who lose many of their previously held rights become aggressive or depressed.

Dean presents with typical problems after TBI, including impaired social judgement, poor conversational skills and disinhibition. The clinicians in the brain injury unit have addressed these problems using a behaviourist approach, without examining in detail why they are occurring. Dean's interests and aspirations have been curtailed or blocked completely. For example, he is not allowed to keep track of information in the racing papers (let alone place bets!), but, more importantly, he is not being supported in his plans to care for his child or his dream of opening a garage. He tries to seek agreement from the staff that these may be successful, but this is not forthcoming. This is a common conundrum for clinicians working with people with TBI. Do they protect the client by providing financial management and supervision, or do they give the person autonomy and independence but risk them losing financial security? Finding some middle ground is probably the best option, where the person with TBI has some control over a part of their life, with support from their family or a case worker, but where their financial security is protected in the long term.

At three months post-injury when the report was written, there is a long road ahead for Dean. At this stage it is difficult to predict his particular circumstances in three or five years time, although one could confidently say that there *is* improvement ahead. It seems counterproductive at this early stage for the staff to withhold agreement about possible future outcomes such as caring for children or getting a job. Dean may well be able to care for his child in some capacity; he may get a job in a garage, even if he can't run a business himself. He may be able to live on his own with support at some time in the future. It is my experience that the more often people are told they can't do something, the stronger the resolve becomes to 'prove you wrong' and the less likely they are to engage in their current treatment.

At discharge Dean probably cannot live on his own, care for his child, work or monitor his conversational skills. So clinicians and families face a number of immediate challenges. These include helping Dean to engage in his treatment, to become increasingly aware of his problems so that he can deal with them, and to focus on the small steps that are needed to achieve his longer-term goals. To facilitate this process, however, the people around Dean need to change their attitudes and ideas about him. It requires a paradigm shift both for his mother and for the staff working with him.

Let's firstly deal with Dean's mother. It is common and completely understandable for mothers to return to a protective, caring role following the accident. I worked once with the mother of a severely injured son, who would challenge every clinician about what we were doing and physically stand between us and him. In some cases, she refused access to him altogether. Once he had recovered, and went to work in a car garage as Dean hopes to, she wrote our team a letter explaining how she felt during these early days. She wrote that she felt like a mother elephant protecting her young baby elephant, and it was a deep primal feeling that overwhelmed her. She realized later that this had made it difficult for us when we tried to treat him. In my research work I have seen how mothers talk differently to their brain-injured sons compared to how they interact with their sons without a brain injury (Togher, Hand & Code, 1997). In some cases, mothers spoke to their adult sons as if they were adolescents or children. So what can we do about this? Training parents regarding how they communicate with the person with brain injury may be an option. This can include highlighting awareness of current communication patterns, and teaching collaborative conversational strategies.

Clinicians have a critical role to play in the successful rehabilitation of people with TBI, in terms both of how goals are set and of the style of interactions which achieve these goals. It appears that Dean's interactions with staff were fraught with negative emotion and aggression. The policy of not responding to Dean's disinhibited remarks is a negative response following occurrence of the behaviour. Treatment was described as encouraging Dean to talk about a wider range of topics; however, one could ask, what is the point to these conversations? Why would Dean find them motivating or interesting? How would these conversations relate to his life after discharge from the ward? It is one of the difficult realities that clinicians who work with people with TBI often come from a different social demographic, and therefore the kinds of interactions they view as 'appropriate' can seem very different to the client. These differences can lead to the person with TBI being penalized or left out of interactions when their conversational interactions do not match with what is considered appropriate behaviour. One solution to this is to encourage people with TBI to interact with their peers (with and without TBI), who can provide the context for the use of humour, irreverent topics, joke telling and collaborative discourse opportunities that are not available in interactions with clinicians (Togher, Taylor, Smith & Grant, 2006).

Another solution is to provide positive antecedent supports with the goal of providing Dean with a satisfying life (Ylvisaker, Jacobs & Feeney, 2003). Strategies could include helping Dean to understand and then providing support to achieve his needs, engaging him in meaningful activities and settings, and allowing him to set his goals, advocate for himself and help create supports with the clinicians. For example, Dean wants a caring role with his son. In discussion with Dean's and Maria's parents, this could be a focus of treatment, whereby he is helped to interact with his son and learn parenting skills. Similarly, his interest in racing might not be the problem his mother thinks it is, if it is introduced within treatment as a highly motivating topic. By focusing on topics and issues that are of interest to Dean, the disinhibited comments and poor topic choices may reduce in frequency, simply because he now has something he is interested in talking about.

Perhaps a more overarching solution to the problem of Dean's so-called inappropriate conversational topics or challenging behaviour is to examine the values clinicians bring to their work when making clinical decisions. One would expect that when a clinician has negative emotions during interactions with a person such as Dean it will deleteriously influence their future interactions, by making them less conversational. Clinicians might shift their treatment focus to tasks they can control, such as controlled discourse tasks that may have little relationship to everyday communication. Clinicians might limit the length and nature of interactions, or, as in one case I reported some years ago, engage in a series of challenging comments and overlapping utterances to maintain control over the interaction (Togher et al., 1997). Experiencing conflict in interactions with clients has other ramifications for clinicians, such as a reduction in job satisfaction and ultimately possible burnout. Making values such as respect, equality and participation in treatment explicit both to clinicians and to organizations and rehabilitation teams as a whole may be one way of circumventing these problems (Byng, Cairns & Duchan, 2002).

The key issue raised by this scenario, however, is the devastating loss of control after TBI. In the effort to protect the person, withdrawing rights may appear a reasonable response; but the implications can be far-reaching for treatment outcomes. The challenge is to achieve a balance between helping the person with TBI actively contribute and ensuring that no harm is done to them or others. Respecting their needs, wishes and aspirations for the future and including these in the clinical process, even if some are longer-term, can help people like Dean become more active participants in their rehabilitation and consequently in their new life.

Leanne Togher, Senior Research Fellow, National Health and Medical Research Council, Faculty of Health Sciences, The University of Sydney, Australia

Commentary on Scenario 5.2

Lyn Turkstra

The case of Dean Taverner is typical of what one might encounter in a sub-acute rehabilitation setting. It appears that Dean has not fully recovered insight into his deficits, yet his verbal skills and mobility allow him to act on his intentions. The main ethical issues surround the conflict between the opinions of his therapists and caregivers about what's best for Dean, and Dean's right to make decisions affecting his own future. The case is further complicated by the need to consider the interests of a minor child, with whom Dean has an important relationship.

In this case, the most ethical course is to consider the legal rights of the different parties so that Dean's rights are not abrogated by well-intentioned caregivers and staff and to ensure that the rights of staff, caregivers, the minor child and other patients are protected. That is, while everyone but Dean might agree that he's best served by not being allowed to place bets or live independently, it is unethical to ignore Dean's rights as an adult without determining that he is unable to make those decisions. At the same time, it would be unethical to send Dean home to live with his mother without any supports, given the health status of Mrs Taverner and the possible pre-existing conflicts between Dean and his mother. Mrs Taverner also might fear that she will need to provide financial support for Dean if he loses money gambling. These competing interests must be considered from both an ethical and a legal perspective.

It appears that there has been no formal determination of Dean's competence to make medical, legal or financial decisions. This is common in brain injury rehabilitation, particularly in the early stages post-injury. When the individual is unconscious or clearly impaired – such as when he or she is in minimally conscious state – there is no question that the hospital must turn to legal surrogates to make emergency medical decisions. At some future time, the individual may clearly be able to make decisions, and there may be no debate about his or her competence. The challenge is in the middle, when the patient is conscious (in terms of level of arousal) and generally aware of his or her surroundings, yet not able to reason effectively. This is when reference to legal guidelines is most helpful. It is particularly relevant here because Dean appears not to have had the best reasoning ability prior to the injury, a factor which is likely to influence the motives and goals of caregivers. There also may be a strong motive to let Dean do what he wants, to avoid conflict, given that he has been verbally and physically aggressive when others disagree with him.

The determination of competence has become a central issue in the care of individuals with acquired cognitive impairments. Reid-Proctor, Galin and Cummings (2001) published a useful review of this topic in patients with frontal lobe injury, and the information is relevant to Dean's case. First, they noted that the law assumes that an adult is competent unless it is proven otherwise. Thus, in the absence of a competence determination, it is both unethical and illegal to prevent Dean from pursuing his goal of independently owning a business, however unrealistic it might be, unless he breaks the law or poses a danger to himself or others. It is also both unethical and illegal to refuse to provide assistance for which Dean might be eligible, on the grounds that he is unlikely to be successful: that is, to discriminate against Dean on the basis of his disability.

The difficulty in making decisions about Dean's future is compounded by the fact that we have relatively little empirical data on which to base predictions of outcomes like business success. Our experience might suggest that Dean will fail, but that is not evidence. Likewise, our social value judgements might lead us to discourage Dean from perseverating on a limited range of topics, but if that is what Dean wants and he is competent to make that decision, is it ethical for the clinician to try to change his behavior? The therapist might feel an obligation to help Dean practise social skills that could improve his social inclusion, but if Dean decides that this is not a problem it would seem unethical to pursue this avenue of treatment.

As Reid-Proctor and colleagues (2001) note, the relation of cognitive functioning to competence is only beginning to be studied, and that has been primarily in individuals with dementia. Existing clinical tests of decision making lack predictive and ecological validity, so it is not clear how one would predict Dean's community behavior based on his test and therapy performance. While many individuals with frontal lobe injury have difficulty in unstructured settings beyond the clinic, many others benefit from a return to their familiar routines and environments. Thus it would be unethical to base long-term decisions on Dean's current neuropsychological test results alone, in the absence of empirical evidence that these tests predict everyday decision making.

A second point raised by Reid-Proctor and colleagues (2001) is that legally, unless an individual has been deemed incompetent, that individual has a right to information that will assist in decision making. In this case, one might ask if Dean has the right to know that Mr and Mrs Bianchi might contest his custody of Kyle. This seems to be more hearsay than fact and might evoke aggressive behavior from Dean toward his late partner's parents. Also, much could change over the next few months. As Kyle is currently living with his grandparents and there is no decision to be made at this time, there does not appear to be an ethical imperative to tell Dean about this rumor of a possible future action.

One ethical issue with a clear answer is whether the therapist should tell the police about Dean's confessed pre-accident marijuana use. This is answerable on empirical grounds. The therapist has determined that Dean has memory problems and that his recall for events up to one week pre-injury is unreliable. Thus, Dean is as likely to have heard this story from someone else as he is to have recalled it from personal experience. The therapist would be unethical if he or she reported it to the police as fact. It is common for individuals with declarative memory impairments to incorporate information told to them by others into their personal event narratives. Many individuals with TBI have impairments in source memory: that is, they are less able than their peers to differentiate personal experience from what they heard, read or saw someone else do. Confabulation also is fairly common with an injury such as Dean's that involves severe bilateral frontal lobe injury, so it is possible that this story is a fusion of Dean's previous life experiences and bits of information related to the accident. It would be unethical for the therapist to report this to the police.

Perhaps the most important factor in this case is time. Dean is in the very early stages post-injury, when expectations for formal logic are far lower than they will be in the future. Given the well-documented trajectory of recovery of intellectual function after TBI, it would be unethical to make long-term decisions such as child custody or independent living based on Dean's current status. If Dean is in fact deemed incompetent to make financial or legal decisions, it might be more acceptable to him if it is established that this is on an interim basis pending ongoing evaluation of his competence.

Lyn Turkstra, Associate Professor, Department of Communicative Disorders, University of Wisconsin-Madison, USA

Discussion

The clients in both scenarios in this chapter are at transition points in the therapy process. Julianna is to be put on review after a (brief) period of therapy. Dean is being transferred to another service following a stay on a rehabilitation ward. The commentators' views on the way in which Julianna's transition has been handled are discussed below, together with the potential conflict of interest faced by her therapist. Julianna's husband has taken a role in advocating on her behalf and we discuss this, as well as the external control taken by various people in relation to Dean.

The manner in which Julianna's therapy has been terminated is described by Togher as 'a surprise to Julianna and her husband' and by Cruice as an 'abrupt end of speech and language therapy treatment . . . for which [Julianna and Dr Jankowski] were unprepared'. Not surprisingly, both commentators view this state of affairs as unsatisfactory. From the perspectives of patient and carer it is difficult to think of an aspect of therapy imbued with greater significance than termination of treatment, representing anything from achievement of whatever outcome they had in mind at the commencement of therapy to forced acceptance of the unachievability of those aims. It is, as Togher writes, 'an increasingly vexing and problematic issue for speech pathologists around the world' in light of increases in financial pressure and expectations of healthcare consumers. Considering this, it is surprising that it has not been the subject of widespread discussion or research. A search through the indexes of medical ethics books and the keywords of medical ethics journals produces nothing of relevance to Julianna's situation. To some extent this is also true of SLT. 'Compared to the vast amount of research on how to assess and treat people with aphasia, the issue of how to stop treating them remains underexplored' (Hersh, 2003, p. 1008), and Hersh has contributed to attempts to rectify that situation. It seems reasonable to assume that the lack of discussion in the medical ethics literature may reflect the fact that the dissolution of (potentially) long-term relationships in medical practice is not the significant issue that it is in therapy, whereas the paucity of literature on discharge in SLT is more likely attributable to the fact that the profession is only just starting to address it in detail.

From interviews with SLTs, Hersh (2003) identified 19 strategies that therapists use in dealing with discharge, subdivided into five categories: wait-and-see, negotiation, preparation, separation and replacement. The suggestions by the commentators as to how discharge could have been handled better for Julianna pick up several of these strategies: discussion of goals, raising the issue of discharge in advance (negotiation strategies), reinforcement of functional goals (preparation) and transferring clients to another service (replacement), in this case the Stroke Group. In fact, central to the recommendations for better handling of discharge is the idea that it should be a process rather than an event. In addition, it should involve the client and carer throughout, so as to be jointly owned and transparent; in Hersh's (2003) words 'not simply a passive drift to independence but something involving planning, effort, and negotiation, that occurs over a period of time' (p. 1008).

The gap between best practice for Julianna and the actual situation she finds herself in can be viewed from an ethical perspective. Although the gross outcome – discharge from the service – might in effect be the same either way, at stake here is Julianna's (and her husband's) sense that they have been prepared for the decision and that they have received from the service the (beneficent) best that can be managed in the circumstances. Thus Julianna and Dr Jankowski could reasonably have expected a much higher degree of involvement in the process and thus a greater sense of control. It may in fact be the case that Ms Sharma feels she has undertaken some negotiation of the therapy and discharge processes, but what is of greater importance here is Julianna and her husband's perception of that negotiation.

Given that therapy for Julianna is being terminated (or at least put on hold), what are the alternatives? One suggestion in Scenario 5.1 is for her to attend a stroke group, but Dr Jankowski's reaction to this is less than positive. Putting aside temporarily the issue of his advocacy role, the other alternative proposed here is for Ms Sharma to provide therapy on a private basis.

Dr Jankowski's invitation to Ms Sharma to consider providing therapy privately '[s]hould it prove impossible for the speech and language therapy service to reconsider the decision to terminate therapy' raises an obvious potential conflict of interest for Ms Sharma. On the one hand, she could perhaps provide some benefit to Julianna through the continuation of therapy; on the other, she stands to make a profit from a decision – possibly her own – not to provide that therapy via the statutory service. Paring this back to the ethical basics, Beauchamp and Childress (2009) describe the (theoretical) obligation in relation to fidelity towards patients as requiring that 'the professional effaces self-interest in any situation that may conflict with the patient's interests' (p. 311). This obligation is generally not seen in such absolute terms (e.g. doctors are not viewed as being obliged to work in the middle of dangerous epidemics at risk to themselves, though they may be applauded for doing so). The situation for Ms Sharma is complicated by the fact that Julianna's interests may coincide with her own in one way (potential continuation of therapy) but collide in another (unnecessary payment). Guidance from the UK Health Professions Council is representative of one approach to this issue: 'Any potential financial reward should not play a part in the advice or recommendations of products and services you give' (Health Professions Council, 2008, p. 14). This is somewhat different to the approach taken by ASHA (2008a), which asserts that 'once people are fully informed of the choices available to them, they have the right to choose whether and from whom they wish to obtain professional services for their communication problems' (p. 3).

The basis for the decision to terminate therapy is not clear from Dr Jankowski's letter (hence some of his confusion). If Ms Sharma has decided that Julianna can no longer benefit from therapy, she would clearly be on unsafe ethical ground in then going ahead and providing the (unnecessary) therapy privately. If the decision arises from a managerial policy, Ms Sharma is still in an awkward ethical position. She is herself not entirely separate from the managerial policy since she presumably has input to policy decisions. If for some reason she does not have input, she will still be open to the perception that she does. This is not to say that public and private approaches to therapy cannot coexist. Togher describes a situation in which a therapist might take on private work from another health district, and Cruice suggests that Ms Sharma should provide Dr Jankowski and his wife with contacts for a number of private therapists. Moreover, what is deemed acceptable practice may vary considerably with context. For example, in Australia and South East Asian countries, where the number of public health positions is limited (so a country town might have only two days a week covered at the local hospital), it is not uncommon for the SLT in the public sector to also run a private practice and see clients not able to get into the public service because of waiting lists or prioritisation. To some extent at least, this means that conflicts of interest are in the eye of several different beholders.

Advocacy and empowerment

We return now to the question of advocacy. Togher sees Julianna as being 'lucky that she has an intelligent advocate who can write a letter of complaint about her discontinuation of treatment'. This is certainly true, given that Julianna would have found it that much harder to register a protest had she been on her own. Chances are she might not have attempted it. But the inclusion of someone in the role of advocate in the therapy relationship brings its own challenges. Ms Sharma will most likely have set out with a working assumption that Dr Jankowski is an appropriate and sensitive representative of his wife's interests, and she appears to have made efforts to include him in the therapy.

Every so often therapists encounter situations in which a carer or representative is clearly not acting in a client's best interests. Evidence of physical or psychological abuse serves as an example. Most of the time, however, deviations from what the therapist perceives as the client's interests are not as dramatic as this. Parents may not bring their young child for therapy (Chapter 6) or a care worker may obstruct (or, more subtly, not facilitate) a disabled person's access to a sex life (Chapter 4). Here, Dr Jankowski expresses the view that attendance at a stroke group is not appropriate for his wife and '[t]here is a concern that the letter might reflect only the husband's wishes, as well as a concern that he may be overprotective or even controlling in making decisions about what could be helpful for his wife' (Cruice). If in doubt, Ms Sharma is under an obligation here to check the decision directly with Julianna while keeping an eye on Dr Jankowski's sensibilities.

In fact, this obligation is symbolic of a much deeper ethical and cultural issue. Without wishing to burden Ms Sharma with responsibility for the philosophies underpinning aphasia services worldwide, the way that she solicits Julianna's views on attendance at the Stroke Group is representative of wider issues of access and inclusion and the search for what Pound et al. (2007) describe as 'a less paternalistic system of health delivery' (p. 24). This has its roots largely in the disability rights movement and has resulted in a greater focus in official policy documents on the involvement of service users in decision making, though Pound et al. also recognise that 'the means and mechanisms of translating policy rhetoric into everyday practice are less explicitly articulated' (p. 24). Cruice (2007), in a discussion of various types of access, employs an image from physical disability in which someone in a wheelchair has access to a building but only by going past the bins and in via the back door. She ponders the feelings that this might engender, some of which might be close to what Julianna is feeling about access via her husband's letter-writing. For Julianna to have what Cruice describes as psychological access, she needs to feel not only that she can express her views but also that she has a right to express those views. Given that Julianna is likely to already feel disempowered by the need to have her husband write a letter for her, it is incumbent on a therapist (whose expertise lies in the field of communication impairment) to demonstrate the highest levels of inclusive practice to assist Julianna in regaining some control.

In the UK the development of more inclusive practice for people with acquired communication disorders has found its most conceptually solid and (as a result) high-profile expression in the work of Connect, a communication disability network. In the article cited by Togher, Byng et al. (2002) set out both an argument for developing 'ways for professionals to become aware of the moral, value-based underpinnings of their practice' (p. 97) and a set of specific values espoused by Connect. One example of how the values are converted into practice is that students arriving to start clinical placement take part in a meeting where personal and organisational values are discussed, together with explanation of how these might relate to their work as SLTs. For such a simple piece of organisational practice, this has a distinctly arresting quality. How many other organisations have a similar practice? Probably relatively few, and most probably not those that have been providing services to Julianna and Dean. Yet this has enormous potential for helping students (and indeed everyone involved) to frame and revisit the core of their work.

Autonomy and control

As with Julianna, the issue of control – or, more saliently, loss of control – is also central to the situation described in Scenario 5.2. Here we find Dean some three months after a significant brain injury, confused, angry and a handful for staff and the other patients on the ward. As Turkstra notes, although Dean has not fully recovered insight into his deficits, 'his verbal skills and mobility allow him to act on his intentions', a powerful combination which presents Dean and those around him with a number of challenges. A key feature of this situation, as described by Togher, is that he has undergone a radical change from being an independent person to losing control over his most basic rights. Against a background of cognitive changes and in the context of highly charged emotional circumstances (in relation to the key people in his life), Togher notes, 'It is little wonder that people with TBI who lose many of their previously held rights become aggressive or depressed.' This situation is further complicated by the issue of time, in that Dean is at a relatively early stage post-injury and the course of recovery is by no means predictable. Dean's loss of control over so many aspects of his life presents the people handed (or perhaps 'landed with') that control with some fundamental ethical decisions as to what they do with it, and of course how Dean can be helped to regain the control he has lost. And so we arrive again in the realm of one of the central tenets of modern (healthcare) ethical thinking, autonomy. In particular, we arrive at the issue of Dean's right to make autonomous choices that other people may disagree with.

Dean is past the point (coma or a state of significant post-traumatic amnesia) where it is relatively uncontroversial for decisions to be taken on his behalf. When Dean's situation is more stable, it may be appropriate for a formal determination of his ability to make decisions to be carried out, though this can only realistically apply to the major medical, legal and financial decisions that people take in their lives. The legal process is not, for example, likely to apply to Dean's desire to gamble (though it may restrict his access to funds) and will certainly not apply to his selection of conversational topics. Both these stages (the first, where determination of competence is impossible, and the second, following formal determination) have ethical ramifications, and it is of particular note that competence is often conceptualised nowadays as applying to specific decisions or areas of life rather than being a blanket designation. The situation here presents us with the ethical questions that arise where formal determination of capacity cannot be undertaken.

In the current situation there are many areas where the hospital staff (and Dean's friends and relatives) can either support or restrict Dean's autonomy. Even in apparently straightforward clinical decisions about how to work on conversational topics, the balance of autonomy is delicate. Is Dean's autonomy increased by supporting his choice of conversational topic or is there any legitimate scope for attempting to render his conversation more 'acceptable' to other people? Both commentators come down in favour of the former, partly to help engage Dean with the therapy process and partly to respect his autonomy. Although 'our social value judgements might lead us to discourage Dean from perseverating on a limited range of topics, ... if that is what Dean wants and he is competent to make that decision, is it ethical for the clinician to try to change his behavior?' (Turkstra). In previous work Togher (2001) has drawn attention to asymmetries that can develop in interactions involving people after TBI, in the conversational roles that are allocated to them. She states that one way to begin to address the goal of removing inequalities is 'to provide access to prestigious discourse types' (p. 144). At its simplest, this may mean providing opportunities for Dean to act in the information-giving role in conversation. Just to complicate matters further, the approach championed by conversation analysts, i.e. that conversation is a joint, co-constructed endeavour, suggests that Dean's autonomous right to choose his conversational topics is matched by his interlocutors' right to ignore him should they see fit.

Another issue raised in Scenario 5.2 and the commentaries is the extent to which therapy should engage with Dean's plans regarding his son, Kyle, in the light of possible moves by Kyle's grandparents to limit Dean's access. Turkstra feels that there is no imperative to inform Dean of what are currently unconfirmed plans regarding Kyle. This general subject area is also discussed by Colicutt McGrath (2007) in her book on ethical practice in brain injury rehabilitation. She supports the use of 'vague' answers to questions about horizon goals, i.e. those that are some way off in the distance. She argues that although this sort of response to clients' questions may feel dishonest (and therefore unethical), it may in fact be a good ethical response in relation to such goals. Long-term outcome is inherently uncertain and horizon goals only come into focus as we get closer to them, so anything other than a vague answer might in fact be inaccurate. Togher applies the same reasoning to this issue as to discussion of cars and horse racing. Dean's plan is to look after Kyle and that is what he wants to talk about. It may be appropriate for the SLT to introduce factors in relation to Kyle for Dean to consider as the situation develops, but ultimately Dean needs to drive the plan and the choice of topic.

Togher sees the positions described above as requiring a paradigm shift by staff to better support Dean's rehabilitation. Underlying this need for a shift may be the associated need for staff to set aside their own judgements of some of Dean's behaviour. He has contributed – possibly under the influence of drugs – to the death of his child's mother but still makes disparaging remarks about her. He also makes sexually inappropriate remarks to the people trying to help him, not an intrinsically attractive quality. It is important to recognise that, for some staff at least, the ethical imperative (here taken from the UK Royal College of Speech and Language Therapists Code of Ethics) 'to refrain from discrimination on the basis of age, cultural background, gender, language, race, religion, or any other consideration' (RCSLT, 2006, p. 11) may make significant demands on their powers of empathy, but that is exactly what is required of them in their professional role. However, they also have an accompanying right not to tolerate personally offensive or threatening behaviour and language.

Summary

In this chapter on acquired communication disorders we have looked at a variety of issues, including termination of therapy, advocacy and empowerment, and what happens when people lose (or are perceived to have lost) control of their lives.

The subject of discharge from therapy has received relatively little attention, despite its potential effect both on people who have taken part in therapy and on their carers. What evidence there is suggests that successful termination of therapy needs to be viewed and undertaken as a negotiated process so that it becomes a natural outcome of therapeutic work rather than an unexpected surprise.

The loss of control occasioned by a sudden event such as stroke or traumatic brain injury leads to an inevitable transfer of control to other people, especially in the acute stage. That transfer of control can take multiple forms (speaking for, deciding for, withholding information from) and confers powerful ethical obligations on the recipients. Clinicians may need to achieve a delicate balance between wishes stated on behalf of a patient and what they perceive the patient may actually want. Broader social movements focused on empowering people who have acquired a communication difficulty are beginning to help address the imbalance in control at a deeper level.

6 Paediatric speech and language disorders

Lindy McAllister, Caroline Pickstone and Richard Body

Introduction

The UK government recently undertook a comprehensive review of services for children and young people with speech, language and communication needs (Department for Children, Schools and Families, 2008), known generally as the Bercow Review. Although the report's detailed findings apply specifically to the UK, the overall conclusions can reasonably be taken as relevant to children everywhere. Primary themes of the report highlight the importance of (a) communication as the key to life, (b) early identification and intervention of speech, language and communication needs, (c) services designed around the family and (d) joint working across different agencies. The conclusion about current services (in the UK at least) is that they are characterised by high geographical variability and a lack of equity. For the considerable number of SLTs working with children these conclusions will come as (a) an affirmation of the importance of what they do and (b) no surprise.

The variation across age groups and conditions that come under the label of paediatric speech and language therapy serves to illustrate the breadth of the field. A two-year-old child with a cleft palate, a five-year-old with developmental dyspraxia and a 10-year-old with specific language impairment bear little resemblance to each other. According to a systematic review of prevalence studies of speech and language delay carried out by Law, Boyle, Harris, Harkness and Nye (2000), on average 5.9% of the population of children between the ages of two and five have some level of speech and language delay. Trends in neonatal survival rates, hearing screening for neonates, child health surveillance and educational policies mandating inclusive education mean that many children with whom generalist paediatric SLTs work may have complex or multiple impairments. The ethical challenges raised by so-called mild speech and language impairment and the way they are managed are discussed in Chapter 8. In this chapter we focus on relatively complex language disorders.

Scenario 6.1 focuses on the language development of a preschool child living in an area of socioeonomic disadvantage. Numerous studies have identified significant consequences in later life for many of these children, and their numbers are not insignificant. On the basis of a survey of speech and language disability in an area of socioeonomic disadvantage in the United Kingdom, Broomfield and Dodd (2004) estimate an incidence rate of children with speech and language disability of approximately 85,000–90 000 per year across the UK as a whole. The figure for non-attendance of referred children in their study was 15%. The challenge of engaging 'hard to reach' families, who, crucially, have not proactively sought a service themselves, is one that is discussed at various points in the chapter.

Scenario 6.2 in this chapter focuses on autism spectrum disorder (ASD) and a child at the difficult transition between preschool and school. The basis on which diagnosis of ASD is made is the subject of considerable debate, not least because the label encompasses a very wide range of severity, hence the term 'spectrum'. However diagnosis is made, formulations of ASD universally involve difficulty with communication, particularly social use of language, as a central component.

The variations in diagnostic criteria and severity, together with variations in sampling method, make accurate prevalence figures difficult to establish. The UK National Autistic Society combines figures from a UK study by Wing and Gould (1979) and a Swedish study by Ehlers and Gillberg (1993) to arrive at an approximate average figure of 91 per 10,000 (or very approximately one in 100). Debate continues as to the extent to which a perceived increase in incidence over recent years is attributable to greater awareness and more sensitive diagnosis or a true increase in the condition itself.

The children in the two scenarios clearly present very different challenges for the SLT, but there are some commonalities. Speech and language therapy interventions for many children are delivered within multidisciplinary teams. Consultancy models, with associated demands for negotiation and delegation of tasks, are becoming more common. Consequently, in many cases, less time is spent by therapists in direct care and more in managing communication, documentation, training of others, and so on. This style of service delivery through others raises inevitable issues of accountability (Roulstone, 2007). And underlying all work in the paediatric field is the ever-present need for services to modify what they do in order to keep pace with the child's development.

Scenario 6.1

This scenario presents extracts from an SLT's reflective log. Through home visits she has been attempting to engage a family in SLT services for their child with suspected delayed development.

Name: *Della Burgess*

Age: *26 months*

Family: *Mother - Pauline Burgess (age 25). Single parent, though maintains intermittent contact with Della's father. Brother - Patrick Burgess (age 5) (? different father)*

Referral: *Referred by Health Visitor. Concern re. Della's language and general development. Family doctor notes refer to periods of depression over last two years.*

Previous contact: *Speech and language therapy appointment sent. Did not attend. Discussed with Health Visitor. Agreed home visit required.*

Therapist reflective log after four contacts with family

Contact 1

Since Pauline hadn't attended the initial appointment, the Health Visitor and I decided to do a home visit together. We hadn't managed to get any confirmation from Pauline that she would be at home and there was no answer when the secretary rang to check.

It took us a while to find Pauline's house as there was no number. The house itself - and in fact the whole street - looked pretty run down. There was an old fridge in the front garden and the grass looked as if it had never been cut. The doorbell didn't work and when we knocked on the door the dog inside seemed to be hurling itself around in a frenzy. After a while we went round to the back and Pauline came to the door. She was still in her dressing gown and looked as if she'd just woken up but she seemed happy enough to let us in.

We all went into the front room, where Della was sitting on the floor, watching the television and filling an empty yoghurt pot with wax crayons. She was leaning against the dog, which was about twice her size. Pauline looked stressed but talked openly about Della. She agreed that Della wasn't talking much but was more concerned about her tantrums. She said Della would often 'go off on one' at the shops and she felt that Della was winding her up deliberately. She didn't dare take Della to the new playgroup in case she played up when they were there.

At this point Della got up and started tugging at Pauline's dressing gown. She said something to Pauline that I couldn't understand but Pauline seemed to and got her a drink and a bag of crisps from the kitchen. Della sat next to Pauline on the sofa, seemingly unconcerned about us being there.

I asked Pauline whether she got any support from anyone. She said she didn't really have any friends and was too busy trying to deal with Della's behaviour to think about making new ones. Pauline's mum lives just round the corner. Pauline told us that her mum takes Della off her hands sometimes to give her a break but also said that she feels criticised because her mum has different views on how to manage Della's behaviour. Pauline said there was also someone from the council who came round and talked to her about managing her money.

We talked about Patrick - Della's brother - who has been at school since September. His teacher had said that he hadn't really settled in and Pauline felt they were saying she should have done more to help him before he started.

I'd taken along a teaset and a small doll. When Della had finished her crisps she started to show an interest in the toys. She offered the dog a cup of tea and then offered one to Pauline, who joined in but looked embarrassed. Della played for about five minutes and used several single words (some intelligible in context) but didn't join words together. When I started to pack the toys away she shrieked and banged her heels on the floor.

We talked to Pauline about Della's development. Pauline said she thought there was nothing wrong with Della's talking but she was difficult to handle. Obviously we needed to do some more assessment and so we arranged that I would visit her again to start that process. Pauline seemed happy with that arrangement although she was distracted by Della, who was difficult to placate. We left to the sound of the dog barking at a noise from outside and I felt awkward leaving Pauline with a difficult situation to handle.

Contact 2

This was the follow-up session and I went on my own. Mrs Burgess (Pauline's mother) arrived at the same time as I did. She'd got some clean washing with her. She made us all a cup of tea and then sat in the kitchen with hers, watching us in the front room. I made a point of saying I'd like to talk to her and Pauline together at the end of the session. Mrs Burgess didn't respond to this.

I'd taken some standard play materials and I encouraged Pauline to play with Della so that I could observe. I made several suggestions. To each one Pauline said, 'Yeah, I do that.' When Della reached for the doll, her grandmother called from the kitchen, 'Make her ask for it.' Pauline tried this but it set Della off screaming and in the end she handed it over.

At the end of the session Mrs Burgess chose to stay put and join in the conversation through the open door. At one point she laughed and commented that nobody had ever come round to teach her how to play with her kids. 'We didn't want to see a speech therapist,' she said, 'it was the Health Visitor's idea. Anyway Della will have to start talking when she gets to nursery.' Pauline had seemed reserved throughout the session and didn't really say much at the end.

The picture emerging by the end of the session was of a child with some language delay and behaviour difficulties. Her mum didn't appear to have many strategies to deal with either, or much general support. The level of language stimulation in the home was pretty low, and given Patrick's history there was an overall sense that this situation would not turn out very well if there was no intervention.

However, I got the impression that Pauline felt therapy should involve getting Della to say things.

Contact 3

Home visit. There was no answer when I knocked on the door. The dog barked for ages and I thought I could hear Della crying. I tried ringing Pauline's mobile but couldn't get a connection. My sense was that there was somebody in the house but no-one answered.

Contact 4

I rang Pauline at home and she answered. She was very evasive and said she would ring me back when she had time. I tried again a week later but got no answer. After six weeks there had been no further contact from Pauline. I organised a meeting with the Health Visitor and managed to make contact with the person from the council, who turned out to be a social worker. She felt it was important that we did not break contact altogether and offered to work with the family under my supervision. The Health Visitor offered to help with this. This is where we've got to so far and seems like it might be our only option.

Commentary on Scenario 6.1

Linda Hand

How much should we persevere when people do not seem to want us? The easy way to deal with this scenario is to call upon one of those decision trees wherein 'being wanted by the caregivers' is an early decision point in the delivery of services. There is always too much for an SLT to do, too many cases to see, and if our services are not wanted, then we should not be involved. This judgement can be backed up by evidence that children make more progress when their caregivers are positive about speech and language therapy and engaged in the process (Gillam & Gillam, 2006). Therefore, spending the time and effort that would be needed on Della may be a waste of precious resources; we may be denying services to another child who may make more progress. It is also reasonable to say that clients have a right to privacy ('Don't come knocking on my door; leave me alone unless I seek you out') and a right to make their own decisions about what is right for their children. We do not have the right to impose our judgements. Therefore one logical and perhaps ethical decision here is to withdraw.

The big problem with this line of argument is that the child is the one with no say but with all the potential consequences. Is it ethical to leave a child without support that may make a difference to their future? Not according to the United Nations Convention on the Rights of the Child (1989). There are those for whom this point is the overwhelming one, and who would therefore argue that our greatest ethical obligation is to do whatever is necessary to get our services to the child. It is not about the caregivers, it is about the child.

But there is more to this case than that. Both the possibilities above – to withdraw or to persevere – are largely about how to get business-as-usual instigated. Instead, I would argue that hard to reach cases are often pointing out inadequacies in our service, and the ethical response is to take up the points of inadequacy. There are two issues that strike me about this scenario, and these two stem from two interests of mine, namely cultural issues in speech and language therapy and discourse analysis and what it can tell us about what we do.

First of all, the rich description in this scenario shows us that human communication is a complex thing and a socially embedded one. This case is not just about the child. It is about the beliefs and attitudes of both the client-complex (it is not just the child – in this case it is the child-mother-grandmother) *and* the clinician or service. It is also about the resources people have available – time, money, effort/energy and social power – and it is about the interactions that go on in the negotiations of service. My argument is that effective – and ethical – service requires that this complexity be taken into account in speech and language therapy practices.

The messages from mother and grandmother in this scenario are that they did not know or understand, trust or believe in the worth of what the speech and language therapy service did. Most speech and language therapy services (most professional practices, in fact) depend on knowledge, trust and belief in the service from clients as givens. It is not until we confront a lack of such givens that we realise how important they are, and it can be very disconcerting, and confronting, when we don't get them. There is a tendency to blame the client – they are inconsistent, don't fulfil their obligations, and so on. However, the work in recent years on cross-cultural issues in speech and language therapy generally starts from an understanding that there are different knowledges, beliefs and attitudes between clients and clinicians (e.g. Battle, 2002; Isaac, 2002; Roseberry-McKibbin, 1997, 2000). It teaches us that we should not make assumptions or take shared perspectives for granted.

My contention is that the lessons from cross-cultural study should be applied to within-culture practices. We should treat all clients as having no reason to value or understand what we do before we start. We should make no assumptions in *every* case. Therefore we must see our job as informing, persuading, empowering and negotiating with clients, of engaging with what they think and believe, in order to be effective. We must *adapt*, not just persevere-or-withdraw. There is no indication in this scenario of the extent to which this SLT did any informing-persuading-negotiating, but my own research in professional discourses in speech and language therapy suggests it is unlikely to have occurred (Hand, 2006).

How might this adapted kind of practice look, in the case of Della and her family? It won't be one-size-fits-all, and it won't be easy to fit into a decision tree. It might start by the SLT asking the mother and grandmother what they think about Della's language, and then continuing the discussion from their perspective. Or it might start with the SLT saying that 'most people have only a hazy idea of what speech and language therapy is about, so here is a bit of an outline to explain why I am here'. A third possibility is that it might engage directly with grandmother's implied dismissal of 'teaching her how to play with her kids' by saying something like 'you don't seem very happy about that – does this look trivial to you?' A fourth possibility might have the SLT ask them what they are most concerned about and talk specifically about how the SLT can help with that – accepting that this will probably be Della's behaviour. This kind of practice would recognise that starting with an assessment based on play, with all the hidden work that goes into that ('hidden' because effective play-based assessment needs to look easy and effortless), is unlikely to be very effective in this context because parents may not perceive that such an approach provides any benefits additional to what they already do. Similarly, clients have to wait for any conclusions or diagnoses until we have worked through what our results mean, which may be for hours, days or even weeks – so we must actively prepare them to suspend judgement on the value of our method. In this new kind of practice the SLT might raise very early that time and effort from them, the adults, might be involved, and because they might not have this schema for our service in their heads it will take some working through. We need to make clear to the adults involved with the child what is likely to be asked of them and why, and to negotiate out with them whether this is going to work.

There are many more things that might be tried in an adapted practice: degrees of directness or indirectness, of control or of handing over control, of explanation or demonstration, and the many other variables involved in culturally competent practices (see Battle, 2002; Roseberry-McKibbin, 2004). It would try its best to engage the mother and grandmother as partners, at whatever level works for them.

No-one would deny that this is a tall order. But I would argue that our ethical obligation here is to be as *effective* as we can be. To be ineffective is to waste time, money and goodwill, to perpetuate social problems, and to diminish potential. We also lose opportunities to extend our service and ourselves as clinicians. Work in culturally competent practice also consistently indicates that we have to accept that effective practice takes more time (e.g. Cheng, 2000). More time is not a luxury, it is an essential.

The other issue I have with this scenario concerns its discourse. The rich description of this text appears to give observational data about what actually happened, without value judgements involved. However, although overt judgements might not be present, implicit social messages abound. Terms such as 'single parent', '? different father', occurring as they do very early in the scenario, set a tone of social judgement. The observations tend to list negatives: 'did not attend, 'hadn't managed to get any confirmation', 'no answer', 'no number', 'pretty run down', and so on. Discourse analysis of speech and language therapy, although it is fairly sparse, has consistently shown that the work being done by the discourse is not always what SLTs would claim to be doing. For example, speech and language therapy talk mostly dominates the discourse even when the aim is to get the client to talk; negative evaluations of clients in assessments are much more likely than positive ones, even when there is little or no problem, and so on. Less obvious are the omissions of the discourse – there is no indication of what the SLT said and how she said it, as if her contributions had no impact on the scenario (see Kovarsky, Duchan & Maxwell, 1999, for a number of examples and references to this work on discourse in speech and language therapy).

In the case of this scenario, analysis would show that although this SLT might claim that she is not making social judgements, the discourse reveals otherwise.

Our reluctance to examine our own discourses parallels that of the medical field some decades ago, but the significance of the discourse of the professional to the effectiveness of a service is undeniable.

In conclusion, ethical decisions involve not just the immediate factors of a specific scenario, but wide-ranging issues of what a profession could or should be, and a wider social and cultural awareness. They are a healthy impetus to constantly question and develop our professional practices.

Linda Hand, Senior Lecturer, Speech Sciences Programme, Department of Psychology, The University of Auckland, New Zealand

Commentary on Scenario 6.1

Julie Marshall

Della's case is an interesting one, and for many SLTs who work, for example, in large cities in the UK, it is not atypical. The description of Della's family situation, the SLT's responses and the content and style of her reflective log raise many challenging and interesting ethical questions. For many of these there are no clear answers, but, at least by acknowledging and being prepared to discuss them, we can improve our reflective skills and awareness. This in turn may lead to solutions, perhaps agreed by consensus. A number of the issues raised by this case relate to both personal morals and professional ethics, as well as challenging personal and societal cultural values and assumptions. Making some of these issues more explicit may help us to recognise and alter behaviours and attitudes such as stereotyping which can impact negatively on clinical practice. Some of these issues are explored here in relation to Della's situation.

The family situation and their opinions

There are a number of issues related to the family situation and their ideas and behaviour. Firstly, if the visit to Pauline was not previously arranged with her, we could reflect on whether this was appropriate and if an unannounced visit could exacerbate an already unbalanced power situation. For someone who may already feel negatively judged, it may well be difficult to be expected to engage in a (potentially threatening) discussion about concerns about your child when you have just woken up and are still in nightclothes.

What is the professional's role when parents do not share her knowledge and attitudes, for example about the importance of play and its relationship to language development, the relationship between language and behaviour and the appropriate methods of remediating delayed language, etc.?

The role of Pauline's mother leads me to reflect on how health, educational and social care agencies in countries such as the UK often assume that it is parents who are the predominant adults responsible for caring for and making decisions about a child. Across the world there are many different family/community constellations, even where parents are the *legal* guardians of children. It is an ethical challenge to consider how much professionals can or should engage with other adult family or community members as potential decision makers.

We do not yet seem to have reached a consensus on whether, if families do not engage with speech and language therapy, it is their right, or if at some point this becomes a matter of advocating for the child (cf. the United Nations Convention on the Rights of the Child [1989] and specifically the child's right to services such as education and healthcare), or, more extremely, a child protection issue. In reality, decisions about this are probably not simple and remain challenging for the SLT.

The SLT's responses

In terms of the SLT's responses, it is important to consider how to respond to parents' priorities and concerns. With each family we need to decide whether it is our responsibility to encourage or to enforce communication having a high profile. With some families we may choose to prioritise working directly with the child, while other family members are dealing with other issues which have a higher priority for them at that time, and in some circumstances we may consider it appropriate for families to de-prioritise communication. However, these responses need careful consideration because some or all of them may be interpreted by families as being patronising.

Particularly in overburdened services, careful consideration should be given to how much effort professionals can or should make with individual families. SLTs should be clear about where their responsibility for encouraging change and offering support ends and the responsibility becomes that of the family. This is a particular issue where children are concerned, and service providers need to decide if they have a duty to *always* advocate for children who cannot prioritise or access services themselves. Furthermore, professionals should consider how much additional effort they are able and willing to make with and for families who they perceive to be vulnerable and who may find it especially difficult to access services.

It would be beneficial for the speech and language therapy profession as a whole, as well as for individual professionals, to debate how far it is acceptable to go in challenging families' usual patterns of language socialisation and their ideas about remediation for language delay, particularly if a family believes the child will improve without intervention. There is perhaps insufficient evidence to inform professionals about how language socialisation patterns vary as a reflection of cultural norms, and whether particular patterns are more or less successful at supporting children with potentially normally developing language and those with delayed language. If the evidence base is incomplete, professionals may question their right to ask parents to change, especially when it is unclear what the effects may be of using an unfamiliar communication style. This question is part of a wider debate about how much we respect families' different 'ways of living' and raising their children and how much we impose our ideas on them.

Related to the point above, in this particular case, it is important to be clear whether it is that the child's language levels are so far below the normal range to be a cause for concern *per se*, or if it is that these levels are expected to be inadequate *for success in school* (and are these the same?). This raises a wider issue about what are, and who sets, both short- and long-term communication expectations and whether these expectations vary between communities or individuals. The speech and language therapy and teaching professions seldom consider *what* constitutes normal (especially long-term) communication expectations, but rather the focus is on *how* those expectations are achieved. This issue relates to a wider concern regarding whether lower language development norms should be considered 'acceptable' for children living in deprived socioeconomic settings.

When a child has language delay and there seems to be no physical/intrinsic cause, it is tempting to assume that the child's environment is at fault and that it should be modified. However, given the limited evidence base regarding the effects of modification of the child's environment for language remediation, we should be cautious in our advice to families.

Finally, it is interesting to consider whether it is outside the SLT's role to comment on matters beyond communication, such as healthy eating, or indeed whether all health and social care professionals have a public health responsibility.

The practicalities

Given the limited resources available in many countries for health and social care, it is important for professions to debate whether it is reasonable to devote a disproportionate amount of time to families who do not readily engage, such as Della's. This dilemma can be considered in at least three ways. Firstly, it could be viewed as ethically appropriate to engage on behalf of the child who cannot act for him- or herself. Secondly, it could be seen as economically prudent, because if the child's difficulties can be resolved now it may well be less costly than doing so later. Thirdly, this approach could be considered inappropriate because families have autonomy and responsibility for their own children. This is part of a wider debate, touched on above, regarding the extent to which the state should be responsible for children.

Some speech and language therapy services have policies of automatic discharge if appointments have been missed without explanation. This is understandable in terms of running an efficient service, where all available appointments are used, but it is much more difficult where families and their needs are complex. Furthermore, those judgements may change if professionals are aware of other factors which may be affecting parents' abilities to engage with services, for example parental mental health difficulties. Once SLTs have started working with the family, is there a duty of care to continue, regardless of the family's views and engagement, meaning that novel ways to provide services should be considered?

The reflective log

The reflective log led me to think about how, as therapists, we all make judgements about what we experience and what we choose to report. It is important that we scrutinise our judgements and any conclusions that we may draw from them. This becomes even more important when we report our observations to others. Our cultural background influences what we choose to pay attention to and the value we give to that information – and others may not share our perspectives. For example, reporting on the state of Pauline's house and neighbourhood may indicate to some readers concern about Pauline's personal, financial and local resources. Others reading those observations could interpret them as indicating that an untidy garden and an unkempt house would indicate 'negative' child-rearing skills. Conversely, and just as dangerous, would be an assumption that a tidy house and garden are associated with 'positive' child-rearing skills.

In summary, Della's situation raises many complex moral and ethical issues which are relevant to all SLTs and which make our work complex and challenging.

Julie Marshall, Senior Research Fellow, Research Institute for Health and Social Change & Senior Lecturer in Speech and Language Therapy, Professional Registration Department, Manchester Metropolitan University, UK

Scenario 6.2

Scenario 6.2 involves SLT Vesna, who has physically left work for the day but who is still there mentally, reflecting on an encounter in the supermarket with the mother of a former client who has ASD. Vesna now finds herself sitting at home mulling over her past, current and possibly future involvement with this family.

Vesna had been looking for bread when she felt a hand on her shoulder and turned to see Mrs Adams. She hadn't planned on this type of conversation while at the supermarket. On the plus side, at least the opening exchanges of this afternoon's conversation with Mrs Adams had not been quite as uncomfortable as when they had first met nine months ago. On the other hand, the rest of the conversation was pretty awkward. Now Vesna found herself sipping at a large glass of wine, staring into space and pondering what had gone wrong with the family. And what to do next.

Vesna was surprised that Mrs Adams had come up to talk to her; they both had long shopping lists but Mrs Adams seemed very keen to talk. It was only three months since Sam had started school, but quite a lot seemed to have happened. Mrs Adams said that almost from day one she felt she was getting mixed messages from the class teacher and the special needs teacher about Sam's readiness for school. The class teacher apparently seemed anxious about how to manage Sam, and Mrs Adams felt that the school did not really want Sam there. When Mrs Adams had spoken to Sam's new SLT last week, the SLT had told her that she was still having trouble pinning down the class teacher and the teacher aide for training that would help them work better with Sam. The new SLT said she had had limited contact with the teacher aide assigned to assist Sam in the mainstream classroom and in the playground. In fact the new SLT suspected that there was no support provided to Sam in the playground and told Mrs Adams she had heard from other teachers that Sam was not mixing with other kids and was starting to hit out at them. Mrs Adams had been quite frank with Vesna, saying that she was having trouble warming to the new SLT and wondered if she knew what she was doing working with children like Sam.

Mrs Adams said she wished they had never sent Sam to the school. She became quite tearful and asked Vesna if she could help in any way. Vesna had heard herself say, 'I'll see what I can do.' When she got home she realised she'd left her bread behind.

Vesna remembered how ill at ease she'd felt when she first encountered Sam Adams. She'd just arrived at the kindergarten and the staff had asked if she could give her opinion on a child they were concerned about. She already had three children with special needs to see and programming support to provide for the staff working with them. On the other hand, the staff at the kindergarten were very interested in communication and she had developed a good working relationship with them.

Five-year-old Sam had not long started at the kindergarten but was taking longer than normal to settle in. He'd moved from another centre because of behaviour problems. The staff said they'd had little contact with Sam's mother, who seemed anxious if they tried to talk to her.

Vesna had observed Sam in a group activity with two other children, including one of the children she had originally come to see. There were some all too familiar warning signs of autism spectrum disorder: Sam didn't seem to know how to initiate contact with the other children and did not join in with the other children in a tabletop activity. He fiddled around with some pencils while the other children worked together on a puzzle. He said very little and made little eye contact with the other children or the staff member playing with the children. Vesna felt she should talk to Sam's mother about what she'd observed and asked the staff if they could organise it.

Vesna was not sure how she would broach with Mrs Adams what she'd picked up from watching Sam. How do you handle a conversation like that? Mrs Adams didn't know her, didn't know she'd observed Sam and certainly hadn't asked for her advice.

Mrs Adams had been pretty frosty at first but did later say she and her husband found it almost impossible to get Sam to do what he was asked, and that taking him to the shops was a nightmare. They worried that he had made no friends at kindergarten and was never invited to parties or to friends' homes to play. At the end of the discussion, Mrs Adams agreed that Vesna could do an assessment and come to visit them at home.

As a result of the assessment and home visit, Vesna learned that both Mr and Mrs Adams had considerable concerns about Sam's behaviour and management. While they were reluctant to consider that there might be something seriously wrong with Sam, they were keen for support, especially with getting Sam to follow instructions at home. No-one else would look after Sam for them, which meant they were hardly getting out at all together. They were also worried by the fact that Sam was due to start school in six months' time at local primary school down the road but they weren't at all sure that he was ready. Vesna had recommended a multidisciplinary assessment to get a full picture of Sam's skills. That way, she'd told them, they'd be able to identify Sam's strengths and support needs, and obtain a programme of support and interventions that would help prepare him for school entry.

Vesna had been worried all along about whether Mr and Mrs Adams understood the implications of a diagnosis of ASD. They seemed to think Sam would 'come right once he got to school'. She had tried to broach this with them a few times, but the relationship was a bit delicate and they tended to become defensive. Vesna felt that if she pushed it any further they might withdraw from the service.

The Picture Exchange Communication System, visual timetables and other behaviour management strategies that the team had recommended the kindergarten use were adopted, and in that structured environment Sam had made reasonable progress in the six months between assessment and starting school. But six months was not really long enough to gauge if Sam was ready for school and to make good recommendations to help the school settle him in when he started. In addition, the school had little experience in managing children with autism. The team thought he might do better in a special support unit as a way of making the transition to mainstream school. When those concerns were shared with Mr and Mrs Adams, they were insistent that they wanted Sam to start at his local school at the start of the next school year. Vesna remembered the rather unsatisfactory 'handover' with the new SLT who was now to manage Sam at school. She was a relatively new graduate and Vesna had heard that there was not a lot of professional development or support for that team.

Vesna heard the clock chime 7 p.m. and realised she had better get on with preparing the meal; she was having friends over for dinner. She wished she'd remembered to bring the bread home. She set off for a quick trip to the corner shop, hoping not to get caught in any more awkward conversations.

Commentary on Scenario 6.2

Julie Marshall

My heart went out to Vesna when I read this scenario. There are so many issues in here, particularly related to home versus work boundaries, SLTs' loyalties to patients and other professionals, and respecting parents' opinions and ideas (and what happens when they conflict with professional views). Some of these many ethical dilemmas are also raised in the 'hard to reach populations' scenario. Few of the issues raised in this scenario seem to be unique to a child with autism.

A common thread between this scenario and the 'hard to reach populations' scenario is that both are concerned with clients who are children, which adds a level of complexity to relationships, decision making and ethical dilemmas. Young children are not expected or legally permitted to make autonomous decisions about their education or other services they receive and are generally considered to be vulnerable individuals on whose behalf others must act. Furthermore, much of the SLT's involvement with young children is mediated through relationships with others who are responsible for the child, such as parents and teachers. This means, for parents, that their views regarding what constitutes appropriate speech and language therapy intervention are not the only opinions to be considered, because they are made on *behalf* of the child, unlike the case for an adult patient, who usually makes those decisions for him/herself. For example, adults are entitled to decline speech and language therapy intervention. This is less clear-cut when children are involved.

Vesna seems to feel uncomfortable about her previous relationship with Mrs Adams. I wonder if she has really thought about the difference between having misgivings about the relationship and the advice she gave to the family and feeling guilty about it. Perhaps she feels that in the past she did not act appropriately because she had contact with a child without the family having requested it, but in the circumstances she and the kindergarten staff had been concerned about Sam and were acting in the interests of the child by prioritising his rights and needs. Although this may feel uncomfortable, the hope is that she feels that ethically it was the right decision and, although she may have misgivings or feel regretful about it, she should not feel personally guilty. However, it would be worth Vesna finding out the local nursery or health service employer's guidance regarding advice and intervention with children who have not been formally referred to a service.

Similarly, Vesna provided the family with information and services intended to lead them to pursue a particular educational service for Sam. His parents chose not to take that advice and now appear to regret their decision. However, Vesna should not feel guilty because she respected the family's autonomy to choose what was right for them using the information available. This dilemma illustrates the issue raised above, regarding who has responsibilities and rights to make decisions about a child (and the balance of that decision between parents and professionals).

Boundaries between professional work and home life can be particularly tricky. It could be argued that salaried professionals should be allowed to step out of their professional role outside of working hours. Conversely it could be argued that with a professional role comes a responsibility to clients which does not cease to exist outside of working hours. If one holds the former opinion, compromise may still be beneficial when a relationship with a family is particularly challenging, and any opportunity available should be used to build positive relationships. Of course, whatever one's professional view of the boundaries of professional role, that view will not necessarily be supported or even considered by our clients.

Confidentiality and privacy issues are important and relevant when talking to clients outside the workplace. As a general principle, confidential client-based discussions should not take place outside of the workplace, but in this case it was important to balance priorities – was it more important to offer privacy to the service user or to develop a relationship on whatever terms the family offered?

Being put on the spot, particularly about a child who is no longer on your caseload, and about third parties, such as other professionals, is extremely challenging. Should Vesna have taken the opportunity to rebuild rapport with a mother, to develop her confidence in the current SLT, or should she simply have said that she was not allowed to discuss the case when she was not in full possession of the facts? Again, this is an issue for which a clear set of rules does not exist.

Related to the point above, it is relevant to consider how appropriate it is to intervene regarding a child with a communication difficulty who is not on one's caseload. It could be argued that there is a moral or clinical duty to do so if one recognises that the child has difficulties. Alternatively, it could be considered to be more appropriate to leave it to the SLT currently involved with the family. If the former, this further confuses the questions about work and home boundaries. Does Vesna have professional responsibility to support any child who she knows has speech and language difficulties? Having promised to see what she can now do for the mother, is Vesna now ethically obliged to do so? The situation is challenging because Vesna did not have time to reflect before acting. She was caught in a context where she was particularly vulnerable because her priorities and energies were elsewhere, on her private life rather than her work. She would do well to reflect on her offer to help before deciding what, if anything, she could do to help.

A separate dilemma relates to our responsibilities and duties to families if we suspect that they are receiving less than ideal services, as may be the case regarding the support that Sam is receiving at school. Our loyalties could be considered to lie either with our employers and professional colleagues or with service users and their families. Furthermore, even if we choose to act upon our concerns about the level of support, we cannot be sure that intervening in this way would necessarily help this family.

It is likely that some parents may view their child differently from the SLT. Parents may have different short- and long-term expectations for their child, including expectations of communication skills. The dilemma for many professionals is finding a comfortable compromise position (which may vary from family to family) somewhere between respecting and supporting parental views and imposing their own expert opinions. In Vesna's case this matter is exemplified by the discussion about the parents' versus the SLT's views regarding appropriate schooling for Sam. I would argue that it would help to understand this type of difference of opinion by thinking about cultural differences and cultural competence. SLTs and parents may form separate sub-cultural groups, sometimes with different ideas about language development, intervention, education, etc. These differences may be exacerbated when parents and SLTs do not share social, economic, educational, linguistic, religious, etc., backgrounds. It is important to try to understand each other's perspectives and priorities, as well as the expectations of education and society as a whole, in terms of the child as a communicator.

In conclusion, as with many ethical dilemmas, there are no clear answers. However, it is important for SLTs to distinguish between situations for which they need increased knowledge and experience and situations which they handled well but which leave them feeling uncomfortable because there is no resolution that would satisfy all parties.

Julie Marshall, Senior Research Fellow, Research Institute for Health and Social Change & Senior Lecturer in Speech and Language Therapy, Professional Registration Department, Manchester Metropolitan University, UK

Commentary on Scenario 6.2

Linda Hand

This scenario is about the ethical dilemma of responsibility – where does it end? Vesna's behaviour illustrates a very common problem, where the desire to help people, which is what brought most of us in to this profession in the first place, conflicts with the need to know where boundaries are, and how to keep them appropriate.

A superficial interpretation might suggest that Vesna makes a number of mistakes in this scenario. She is guilty of professional interference, by discussing another SLT's case with a parent. Further, she promises things either which she cannot deliver, or which will place her out of bounds with her colleagues if she does attempt to deliver them. If I was the 'other' SLT here and learned about this interaction, my reaction could range from unimpressed to incensed, and the school personnel would probably have similar reactions. Ultimately, Vesna is unlikely to be able to do anything effective, which will leave the parents perhaps worse off than before as their hopes may have been raised by her promise of help. All of this could be classified as unethical behaviour.

On the other hand, Vesna is confronted with a situation where a child and a family with high needs are not getting these needs met. She may be the only person in a position to convey to others what the problem is and to help find a solution. She is in a position of trust and the family are in a position of need – it is equally reasonable to ask if it is ethical to turn your back on all of this.

On the face of it, however well-meaning the second argument, the first would seem more compelling. No matter how much you might feel for people, boundaries need to be understood, or everyone – clients, colleagues and the SLT – suffers. The foundation point is, 'Whose case is this?'

However, to simply suppress the desire to help and plump for the hard-headed approach may not be the answer. It might simply lead to many of us repeating this scenario, because the fundamental problem has not been solved. The conflicting feelings it generates will cause heartache and possibly lead to burnout, an ongoing professional problem. We need a series of ways to think about the issues more deeply.

The rule about not getting involved in anyone else's case is a useful one. However, the idea of the demarcation of work and personal life is essentially a cultural notion. In Australia and New Zealand (and many other places), one of the things that SLTs may need to deal with is that parents from non-Western cultural backgrounds regard it as OK to discuss issues with you wherever and whenever they see you, because that is who you are and they know that about you. It is like the way notions of time vary enormously across cultures, and must be dealt with, not just ignored, if a profession is to be efficient (Roseberry-McKibbin, 2000).

Even where there does not appear to be a cultural difference between the parties, this lesson can help us understand and deal with the issues involved. It would probably be fair to say that the parents in this case don't care about professional boundaries. They are in too much pain, need and anguish to care. We should not assume that there is anything automatically 'right' about demarcations of responsibility, and that everyone will ultimately value them the same way. In terms of the ethical decision Vesna must make, it may lead her to make the issues explicit or at least open to negotiation (such as whether she should discuss the case with them, and if it is OK to do that in the supermarket). This is not unlike the way that family-centred practice suggests decisions should be negotiated rather than just made (see, e.g., Paul [2007, p. 202], who makes it clear that there are many ways that a family-centred approach changes professional practices). At times, parents need to discuss 'inappropriate' issues with us outside our usual professional boundaries. This should not be considered unethical, though it may present a problem if clinicians feel 'on call' 24 hours a day. The problem for Vesna was more that she felt pressured to fix the problem.

A great deal of this scenario and its difficulty is about emotion. The parent's emotions make Vesna uncomfortable; her own emotions about this lead her to potentially poor judgements. We don't particularly like to talk about or deal with emotion in a work context, as another essentially cultural Western notion about professions and professionals is the idea of detachment. There are many writings which discuss the need to remain detached, how it assists functioning and clear thinking, how emotional involvement clouds judgement and muddies boundaries. This is an underlying premise to the idea that ethical judgement is about objectivity. However, it may be not only a cultural notion but also an essentially gendered one. Writers such as Gilligan (1982) and Belenky, Clinchy, Goldberger and Tarule (1997) have investigated how women's ethical judgements differ from men's, including the fact that relationships and their importance figure more and objectivity and abstract principles less than in men's, which nevertheless was (is) viewed as the dominant – or only – point of view. Speech and language therapy is heavily female-dominant, but this does not mean that women's ways of knowing prevail. We need to adjust this balance. It should lead us to talk about the issues differently, and acknowledge and work with a wider set of perspectives as to what the 'right' judgement is. We need to bring emotions and their validity into the equation rather than seek more rigorously to exclude them.

The notion that the division into personal versus professional is a false one is supported in other areas as well. Ethnological approaches suggest that separation into parts obscures an understanding of the whole (Hammer, 1998). Richer views of communication see it as part of the whole person, the person as part of a whole social system (Halliday & Hasan, 1985). Emotion is a significant part of this complex whole. For example, the way emotions are expressed in language leads to whole systems, such as directness, politeness strategies, appraisal systems and many other areas that in speech and language therapy are often termed 'pragmatics' or 'social skills' in communication (e.g. Paul, 2007). Similarly, we know that there are processes of acceptance – the grief process and similar – that relate to families where disability occurs. Then there are the professionals and their emotions, such as compassion and understanding, many of which are of great value to them. We cannot – and, I would contend, should not – box these into a compartment labelled 'irrelevant' or 'to be ignored wherever possible'. Rather, we should find out how to utilise these to the maximum, to make them into positive forces. Valuing her emotional sensitivity to Mrs Adams and recognising the role of emotions in reasoning might have provided valuable resources for Vesna as she thought 'on the spot' about how to manage the interaction at the supermarket, and as she reflected on the incident later at home. She might even have felt there was no ethical dilemma for her at all, that an appropriate and acceptable thing to do was to respond to Mrs Adams' distress regardless of where and when that was encountered.

For example, we could see emotional change in Sam's parents – from resistance and rejection to seeking help, to wanting change – as part of the process, and have ways to react accordingly. We could accept their input and work with it, while still suggesting ways they can continue to develop their thinking and understanding. We should also value the compassion and the empathy in professionals and support it. We should look squarely at gender issues and how they affect the profession. Rather than seeing the dominance of female numbers in speech and language therapy as a weakness, we should exploit its potential to be a strength. There is very little of this idea visible in speech and language therapy at the present time.

The other thing this discussion highlights is the need for more professional education. We can tell students and qualified professionals a 'rule', but if that rule does not acknowledge and allow ways to deal with the conflicting feelings and the social communication dilemma that it causes (e.g. the encounter in the supermarket), then it will leave Vesna and all of us repeating our mistakes. Problem-based learning can be of great help here. It allows us to play out a problem, find a range of possible ways to deal with it, and see what they will lead to. Dealing with these conflicts should also always appear on the continuing education agenda. We need to keep looking at the issues, not assuming that one solution we find will always be appropriate.

Linda Hand, Senior Lecturer, Speech Sciences Programme, Department of Psychology, The University of Auckland, New Zealand

Discussion

Bronfenbrenner's (1994) ecological model of human development provides a useful framework for considering the complexity of ethical issues raised in this chapter, allowing us to frame the children in the scenarios in a social context and to consider ethical theories, individual ethical decisions and their consequences in the complex contexts in which they are located. Children with communication problems can be seen as developing within a series of contexts, each embedded within even broader contexts. In the layer most immediate to the child (referred to by Bronfenbrenner as the micro-system layer) are the child's close family (including in Della's case her grandmother), siblings, friends and others in close caring roles such as nursery staff (in Sam's case). Each further layer represents increasingly wider influences on the child and family. Health, community, social care and educational services and workers comprise what Bronfenbrenner terms a mesosystem which supports children and their families. Outer circles of the model represent the contexts of policy and the philosophy of the broader community, such as the 'health system', the 'social welfare system', the 'education system' and the levels of law and politics which govern provision of these services. For families under stress, due for example to disadvantage or chronic illness, these outer contexts should ideally offer a supportive rather than an obstructive influence. The scenarios and commentaries in this chapter give us cause to consider whether this is in fact the case.

Marshall summarises the issues raised in Scenario 6.1 about Della in terms of the amount of effort professionals should make with an individual family. Where does the professional's responsibility for encouraging change and offering support end and the responsibility become that of the family? If the problem is seen as lying primarily with families who are vulnerable or 'hard to reach', questions arise about how far we should push such families to engage with our services, about who makes decisions for the non-autonomous children involved, how this is done and when. If the problem is seen as lying primarily with the service in that it is not perceived as useful, relevant or accessible by the family and is for any of these reasons difficult for them to make use of, then this raises questions about how services can and should change and the impact on other potential users of our services if resources are disproportionately allocated.

Service delivery

Hand outlines two possible service delivery responses to the situation involving Della and Pauline (Scenario 6.1), namely to withdraw or to persevere. We look first at arguments in favour of each of these approaches. However, Hand also notes that both these responses operate on the basis of 'business as usual'. She suggests that Scenario 6.1 should instead alert us to the fact that this may not be appropriate and that perhaps some change or adaptation to the service is required. In other words, there will need to be changes at the policy level of the mesosystem described by Bronfenbrenner (1994) or at least agreement to change mechanisms of service delivery.

Withdrawing the service
One argument for withdrawing the service might be, as Marshall points out, that significant input can create incursions on family autonomy. She asks how much right professionals have to attempt to change parents' play and communication styles – in essence a large part of their overall parenting style – when the evidence base for making such changes is limited. Such questions, she says, form part of a needed wider debate on respect for families' different ways of living and raising children and on what constitutes acceptable differences. Della's language development may not be much different from that of other children of similar age and background living in similar socioeconomic circumstances. Should we accept lower language levels from such children as an inevitable consequence? At present, after all, Della's language skills do not appear to be a problem for Della herself or for her immediate family.

The SLT in Scenario 6.1 has made repeated attempts to engage Pauline through home visits and telephone contact, but with little success. Sim (1997) discusses what he calls the cardinal considerations that influence allocation of resources in healthcare, sometimes called the three Es: effectiveness, efficiency and equity. If Pauline and her mother will not or indeed cannot engage with the service (despite the SLT's best efforts), it is difficult to argue that speech and language therapy input is being effective and, as Hand says, 'To be ineffective is to waste time, money and goodwill, to perpetuate social problems, and to diminish potential.' If the input is not effective, then efficiency – the most effective input for the least cost – is not going to be a consideration at all and the argument for withdrawing the service (in its current format at least) appears to be supported.

Perhaps not surprisingly, the question of equity – the fair distribution of burdens and benefits – both here and in general raises the most ethical problems (Sim, 1997). Even if Della has greater need than other children, a system of equitable distribution based on equal share would justify withdrawal once she has received the same amount as other people. A system based on need, on the other hand, would justify provision of the disproportionate amount of input highlighted by Marshall.

Persevering with the input

In speech and language therapy practice it is common for some clients or client groups to receive greater input than others. Rowson (2006) discusses the common challenge of inadequate resources to meet needs and suggests two possible options. The first is to allocate a universal level of provision as a priority *before* providing for any greater needs. The second is to allocate based on varying levels of need. According to Rowson these approaches can sometimes be used to complement each other, and speech and language therapy service managers may well endeavour to offer a universal level and yet still allocate resources above this level where additional needs can be demonstrated.

What, then, are the arguments in favour of persevering with input? The ethical argument is often linked to an economic one. For example, we know that unresolved childhood speech impairments can have significant lifelong impacts on educational, social, relational and economic achievement in adulthood (Felsenfeld, Broen & McGue, 1992, 1994). Language impairments in children are also associated with poorer mental health in adolescents and adults (Snow, in press). Adults with communication impairments tend to be employed in lower-status, less well-paid jobs than those without communication impairments (Felsenfeld et al., 1994). It may therefore be an efficient and ethically justifiable allocation of resources to fund continued speech and language therapy input at this stage if it can be shown that it is likely to lead to reduced possibility of these negative outcomes, though this latter requirement is of course a significant challenge in its own right.

Although there is an argument for withdrawing the service to avoid potential interference with the family's autonomous decisions, a counterargument is that a problem may develop later for the larger social units (as highlighted by the Bronfenbrenner [1994] model) of the school and perhaps society at large if Della's literacy and communication problems prevent her gaining financial and social independence. This view suggests that the problem is not just one for Della and her family, because the school will have to address the issue if Della does not have the language skills to access the curriculum. The fact that the school will not be in a position to withdraw its services might be taken as placing an ethical obligation on the speech and language therapy service to prepare Della for school.

A further factor to be taken into possible consideration arises from the manner in which Della's family became recipients of a service in the first place. Whereas the majority of healthcare delivery is predicated on the principle of people seeking assistance for a problem they have identified, the service to Della's family is based on professionals identifying previously unrecognised areas of need. Screening programmes for children are a prime example of this type of provision. With reference to Beauchamp and Childress's (2009) principles, it is relatively easy to argue that the potential harm of bringing to a family's attention a problem they did not know existed might carry with it an increased obligation to do them some good. Thus, once we commence engagement with a vulnerable family, raising awareness and a perception of need, we may be ethically obliged to provide a follow-up service.

Adapting the service

None of the factors outlined above is a serious argument for simply providing more of an ineffective service. The alternative option to persevering with input or withdrawing the service is to adapt the service for people whose needs do not fit or are not met by a standard model of service. So far we have used the language of 'disproportionate input' and 'greater need', but, according to Hand, our 'ethical obligation here is to be as *effective* as we can be', and that may require us to reconceptualise Della's needs as different rather than just disproportionate. It is of significance in Scenario 6.1 that the input as given has clearly not been successful; more of the same would be difficult to justify.

The term 'hard to reach' – used to characterise Della and her family – is widely applied within healthcare to various groups defined by factors such as aetiology (e.g. some areas of mental health), lifestyle (e.g. gang members), ethnicity (e.g. minorities, culturally separate groups) and geography (e.g. those in remote locations), and in some cases all of these combined. While the concept of people being hard to reach is superficially transparent, the terminology is not without controversy since it is potentially stigmatising. Alternative terms such as 'hidden populations' (Duncan, White & Nicholson, 2003) and 'underserved populations' (Kornfeld et al., 1998) are in use, but 'hard to reach' is the most widely used. In its most positive light, recognition of the fact that not everyone views or uses services in the same way can be seen as reflecting a recognition of and respect for diversity of values and lifestyles. In its least positive light it suggests an approach to a population that emphasises its members' shortcomings rather than the potential inflexibility of the service.

Perhaps the key to the ethical considerations involved in adapting the service to Della lies in approaches to different 'hard to reach' groups. For instance, nowadays it would be deemed unacceptable to provide rigid clinic appointments to members of Travelling communities and then discharge them if they do not attend. Some sort of outreach service seems much more in tune with their needs. Although as an individual Della may not have the status of a 'hard to reach' group as such, her requirements for flexible thinking on the part of service providers may not be dissimilar.

Hand suggests that if families are to engage with our services we need to pace our intervention according to the family's level of understanding at the commencement of intervention. This point is illustrated by the fact that Della's mother and grandmother do not know or understand, trust or believe in the worth of a speech and language therapy service. Both Hand and Marshall draw on what can be learned from cross-cultural service interactions, Hand arguing that irrespective of whether an interaction is cross-cultural or not, '[w]e should treat all clients as having no reason to value or understand what we do before we start. We should make no assumptions in *every* case.' She suggests that our role is to inform, persuade, negotiate and adapt, which highlights the importance of the language we use in our discourse with clients and families, a point we return to later in this chapter. The commentators also suggest we consider both the family's priorities at the time of engagement with our services and the assumptions they may hold about our service (and perhaps all professional services). SLTs can be very challenged by trying to engage families who are dealing with alcohol abuse, domestic violence or child abuse as part of family life. Such families may understandably see speech and language therapy as a non-essential need, as a result of which the focus moves to the role of SLTs in broader health promotion, illness prevention and child safety issues as health professionals rather than just SLTs.

Health promotion

Some interventions for children with communication delays who come from disadvantaged backgrounds involve environmental modification to achieve change in language outcomes. Such interventions are often referred to as health promotion, and include provision of information, screening and prevention of difficulties through early intervention. This field presents ethical challenges to professionals (Cribb & Duncan, 2002) for a number of reasons, including the difficulty of establishing exact terminology (what *is* the nature of health?) and the lack of clarity about the aims and hence the outcomes of intervention. As early as 1990, the American Speech-Language-Hearing Association called for clarity and more research to provide evidence that might inform the scope of practice in this area. In the UK, health promotion is now listed as one of 10 key roles for allied health professionals (Department of Health, 2003). Allied health professionals have historically carried out health promotion work either through working on screening and early identification or by working with children and families deemed to be at risk of communication problems based on their family history or environmental circumstances. Recently, such approaches have been nested within wider interventions (such as Sure Start in the UK) to promote improved developmental outcomes for children (Department for Education and Employment, 1999; Department for Education and Skills, 1999). However, it may be that we have to assume a mandate for health promotion work without detailed evidence, because clarity about aims, objectives and outcomes of health promotion has yet to be achieved, the evidence base for such work is relatively limited, and our understanding of potential benefit and harm is similarly restricted.

Responsibilities and boundaries

Responsibilities and boundaries lie at the heart of Vesna's dilemma (Scenario 6.2), as she contemplates her interaction with Sam's mother. As SLTs, do we have a responsibility to advocate for all children with communication and swallowing problems, known or unknown to us personally, on our caseloads or not? Many SLTs will have been in the position of wondering how to respond to the questions of someone at a party whose child has delayed speech and language and who has been searching the internet for information: 'If my child has only 10 words rather than 50, what should I do?' 'Does that mean he's not developing fast enough?' Does Vesna still have a responsibility to advocate for Sam even though he is no longer on her caseload? Or does she, in fact, have a responsibility *not* to advocate for Sam precisely because he is no longer on her caseload? She could discuss Sam and his mother with the new managing agency (the school) and his new SLT, though she runs the risk of estranging them. Or she could ignore the mother's distress and the child's welfare and stay within the generally understood boundaries of what constitutes ethically good behaviour by not even entering into the conversation with Mrs Adams, in the supermarket or anywhere else.

Being in the supermarket places Vesna outside professional hours and location, that is, off duty. Although off-duty responsibilities are widely discussed in medical and nursing texts (e.g. Hendrick, 2000 – such as when a nurse, say, is faced with someone taken ill in the street), the same does not apply to speech and language therapy. Of the codes of ethics discussed in Chapter 2, none gives specific guidance on off-duty responsibilities. Item 13 of the Standards of Conduct, Performance and Ethics published by the UK Health Professions Council (2008) states, 'You must justify the trust that other people place in you by acting with honesty and integrity *at all times* [our italics]' (p. 14), but this is unlikely to make Vesna's position any clearer. Some codes of ethics do have something to say about Vesna's related dilemma, of whether to take a role in the care of someone who is not only not her client but is also now under the care of another SLT. The South African Speech-Language-Hearing Association Code of Ethics (1997) suggests that professionals should not 'supersede' other professionals, though this again offers only general guidance. Codes of ethics also tend towards minimisation of risk – if in doubt, don't do it – and minimisation of risk is a blunt instrument with which to face Mrs Adams' needs.

Despite the lack of clear external guidance, on the surface this is, as Hand notes, a simple problem. Students to whom we have presented this scenario (Scenario 6.2) for discussion respond by treating the issues as black and white. They tend to come to the conclusion that Vesna has been unethical by breaking rules of confidentiality and privacy – holding the conversation in the supermarket – and discussing a client who is no longer hers. It is clear from the scenario that Vesna recognises the less than desirable setting for the conversation, and indeed feels unsure whether she should be having the conversation anywhere. However, as Marshall points out, Vesna prioritises building a relationship with a mother in crisis and responding to that mother's need over a perhaps rigid interpretation of what might be set out in codes of ethics regarding privacy and confidentiality. She responds from the heart, using emotional intelligence to guide her. Hand argues for an increased recognition and valuing of the role of emotion in professions such as speech and language therapy. She draws on literature around the role of emotion and connectedness in women's ways of knowing and thinking (Gilligan, 1982; Noddings, 2003) and suggests this should be a cause for celebration rather than denigration in a profession that has help, care and compassion as core values. Though advocates of the ethics of care have debated the extent to which these views are essentially feminine (and/or feminist), the empathy underlying Vesna's response to Sam's mother is very much in line with this approach (Slote, 2007). This might be seen as a contentious argument by members of professions who privilege scientific rationality in professional decision making.

Hand's commentary provides some useful ways of thinking about boundaries. She sees the demarcation of work and personal life as an essentially cultural construct, and thus contends that our constructions of boundaries and limits to responsibilities are artificial. Attempts to achieve work/life balance tend to include demarcation of professional time from personal time and thus professional life from personal life. Colicutt McGrath (2007) argues that it does not make sense to talk about work/life balance, because 'professional life is not distinct from personal life but is a special domain within it' (p. 53). Robyn Cross et al. (2008) concur with this view, arguing that ethical concerns at work often spill over into the personal domain, causing worry at home about issues at work and disrupting the putative work/life balance.

There is a sense in which professional boundaries are also maintained via the 'detached professional attitude', one argument being that it facilitates greater objectivity on the part of the professional. Colicutt McGrath (2007) argues that professional detachment may in fact be amoral, since emotion and empathy are the foundations of morality. In any event, attempts to draw boundaries around work versus private life may clash with the boundaries perceived by some cultural groups, whose members may 'know us' as what we are professionally and see no boundaries preventing them from approaching us in any setting if they have need of us and our support. As Hand suggests, the insights from cross-cultural studies that can be applied to negotiating boundaries with members of different cultural groups can also be applied to negotiating with clients and families from cultural groups that are similar to or the same as their service professionals.

As things stand, given that Vesna has already had the conversation with Mrs Adams, she might be advised to consider contacting Mrs Adams again to encourage her to raise her concerns with the new school herself.

Best interests

Both scenarios hinge on the issue of acting in the best interests of children. With Della, questions are raised about who to involve in decision making, how Della's best interests relate to those of her family, and what to do if the family appears not to act in her best interests by not engaging with a service (assuming every effort has been made to adapt the service for the family's needs). In the case of Sam, questions about best interests arise from Vesna's early decision to observe him at kindergarten without parental consent, and later to re-enter a relationship with Mrs Adams when Sam is no longer her client. How do professionals make decisions about which situations call for them to act in the interests of the child and about how to act in the interests of the child in ways that are legally, ethically and socially acceptable?

The principles approach and the ethics of care approach present rather different perspectives on these issues. The starting point of a principles approach would be that neither Della nor Sam is autonomous in the sense of making informed decisions, and therefore those decisions have to be taken on their behalf. The ethics of care moves the focus away from the rights of the individual child (as judged by other people) to the intricate network of relationships in which the child operates:

> It is important to recognize children as significant actors within these networks and any judgements of rights, needs or protection must place children within these networks. Failure to do so, by recourse to abstract principles, will result in an impoverished treatment of social networks. (Cockburn, 2005, p. 77)

Baines (2008) suggests that in fact where children are concerned it is difficult to base clinical decisions on the four principles approach since the most important principle – autonomy – is not applicable to 'incompetent' children. Moreover, it is not clear where to turn if autonomy is not applicable, since the interpretation of the child's best interests (in relation to the principle of beneficence) is also challenging. Because children are located within the microsystem of their family and significant others in their lives (Bronfenbrenner, 1994), decisions made for or about children will impact on others. In particular, Baines argues that it can be difficult to identify a child's best interests in relation to those of others in the family, a situation well illustrated in Della's scenario (Scenario 6.1), and that the best *medical* interests may not tally with other best interests (e.g. social interests). Nelson and Nelson (1995) describe this graphically in terms of the ease with which health professionals 'may unwittingly trample on the intricate web of relationships of which families are woven' (p. 3).

Baines (2008) examines the interpretation of children's interests in a way that might be useful to apply in both Della's and Sam's scenarios (Scenarios 6.1 and 6.2). The first standard that might be applied is that decisions should be taken *in the best interests* of the child. Baines suggests that a significant problem with this is that it 'does not recognise the complex way that interests must be balanced within a family' (p. 143). If 'best interests' of one child is too demanding a standard for a whole family to meet, for example because it would significantly reduce time and attention available to other children, then perhaps removal of the word *best* would result in decisions *in the interests* of the child being less of a challenge. Even here, though, family life is often in conflict with the possibility of all members' interests being met simultaneously. A further possible standard is that decisions should be *not against the child's interests*. However, although Della's family's decision not to engage with speech and language therapy might be perceived as against Della's (communication development) interests, it is unlikely that anyone could sustain an argument for Della to be removed from the family. Baines's compromise position takes the form of a standard representing the child's *reasonable* interests.

This hierarchy may prove conceptually useful in ethical dilemmas where there are multiple stakeholders' needs to consider, and when no one course of action can achieve good outcomes for all involved. Baines further suggests that judgements of *reasonable interest* should be based on the standards of the relevant community. Perhaps that would mean that acting against a child's interests would be acceptable if the harms were limited and were justified by advantages to others in the family group (Baines, 2008). Rowson (2006) similarly proposes that situations such as Della's should be addressed by choosing a course of action which goes as far as possible towards meeting the demands of all, even though it might not meet the demands of anyone in full.

Both Hand and Marshall pay attention to the implications of language used by therapists in their interaction, recognising that it conveys subtle messages about the status of the participants and the attitudes of the professionals. This is particularly the case with some of the subtly negative observations of Della's family's lifestyle. In Chapter 1 we highlighted the ethical importance of language and the implications that choices of individual words and phrases can have. The fact that language is such a constant medium of interaction and that SLTs get through thousands of words a day means that these implications can be difficult to spot, much less manipulate, without objective analysis. Antaki (2001) presents a study of interviews with people with learning difficulty, illustrating ways in which the respondents' answers are shaped by the way questions are structured and delivered. The author comments that the episodes 'are wholly unexceptional and would have passed without comment of any sort, had they not become the focus of some careful going-over' (p. 197). The article in question has as its subtitle 'Dissembling Language and the Construction of an Impoverished Life'.

In similar vein, Duchan, Maxwell and Kovarsky (1999) discuss the degree to which people's identity 'is tied directly to evaluative contexts experienced in everyday life' (p. 4) and the view that 'competence judgements pervade, influence, and grow out of ordinary social interactions' (p. 5). These observations are true both of direct interactions and of written materials, where a turn of phrase or a collection of statements can influence the perceptions of, say, the various professionals reading a report.

The fields of conversation analysis and discourse analysis (particularly discursive psychology) are beginning to offer a developing perspective on a wide array of institutional interactions, such as police interrogations (Edwards, 2006) or out-of-hours calls to general practitioners (Drew, 2006), and focus has also turned to the speech and language therapy process (e.g. Gardner, 2006; Horton, 2008; Simmons-Mackie & Damico, 1999). For instance, Simmons-Mackie and Damico (1999) present a description of a therapy encounter characterised by fixed social roles in which 'routinized features of the institution of therapy . . . hinder the enactment of multiple social roles' (p. 332). Despite these observations and the issues raised in the scenarios in the chapter, this 'going-over' of speech and language therapy discourse is by no means necessarily a negative process. It may indeed throw up some insights that are uncomfortable to consider, but it also has the potential to reveal (and thus contribute to the development of) the high levels of interactional skill employed by SLTs.

Summary

Both Scenarios 6.1 and 6.2, their accompanying responses and the discussion of the issues raised in this chapter highlight a number key points in ethical practice with children. Firstly, children are located within a larger web of relationships within their immediate and extended families and communities, and within policy systems, as described by Bronfenbrenner (1994). Because of this, decisions which SLTs might make about service delivery for children have the potential for impact on a large number of people. What might be seen as being in the interests of the child can in some cases run counter to the interests of the family. Acting to ensure the rights of children might erode autonomy for the family. The factors to be weighed are numerous, ethically and legally complex, and frequently unclear. Secondly, economic and ethical arguments intersect in the provision of services for children. The three Es of ethical resource allocation – effectiveness, efficiency and equity – can be applied to decision making about whether to withdraw services from some families, persevere with services as they currently are offered or adapt them. The economics of resource allocation might superficially indicate withdrawal of services from 'hard to reach' families on the grounds of lack of effectiveness and efficiency. However, this may have ethical overtones in terms of obligations to people with greater need and may have implications in terms of greater economic costs incurred later in children's lives.

Boundaries and responsibilities of SLTs also figure in this chapter. Weighing up boundaries and responsibilities causes us to examine core values and beliefs underlying our practice as SLTs. In making decisions about boundaries and responsibilities, consideration from the perspective of an ethics of care may be as helpful in highlighting ways forward as traditional principle-based approaches to ethical reasoning.

Consideration of the major issues identified in this chapter highlights the need to focus as well on the discourse of our practice. The content of what we say to families about our services, the rationales we offer for our opinions and recommendations, and the manner in which we say these things all have ethical implications. Our discourse can affirm or undermine family autonomy and it can engage families with or disengage them from our services.

7 Degenerative conditions in ageing

Introduction

It is customary for chapters on conditions of ageing to set the context by referring to the ageing of the population as a whole. Taking as broad a perspective as possible, figures published by the Population Division of the Department of Economic and Social Affairs of the United Nations (2007) indicate that of the predicted increase in world population by 2050 (some 2.5 billion), half will be accounted for by people over 60 years of age. Moreover, while this represents a tripling of the population over 60, the population over 80 is set to increase nearly fivefold. Clearly over that period there will also be developments in migration patterns from one country to another and in health conditions that are prevalent in old age. Whichever way these developments pan out, it seems that health professionals who work with older populations are unlikely to find themselves short of work.

A number of conditions relevant to speech and language therapy – stroke being perhaps the most obvious example – are more common in older populations than in younger ones. The onset of progressive neurological conditions is also skewed towards the later stages of life (in populations with sufficiently high life expectancy). Here we focus on two such neurological conditions, dementia and Parkinson's disease (PD). Dementia, the focus of the first scenario, is an umbrella term for symptoms arising from a variety of underlying brain conditions. According to the UK Alzheimer's Society (2008) there are over 100 types of dementia, which share the characteristics of being usually progressive and eventually severe. Gradual loss of cognitive and communication function is the characteristic we are most concerned with here. PD, which is featured in Scenario 7.2, is primarily characterised as one of the movement disorders, with four primary symptoms: tremor, rigidity, bradykinesia (slowness of movement) and postural instability. Symptoms of depression and cognitive change also occur, and in some cases PD shares a number of features with some forms of dementia.

Prevalence rates in the UK for dementia are reported as 1:50 at age 65–75, 1:20 at age 70–80 and 1:5 at over 80 years of age, according to the Royal College of Speech and Language Therapists (RCSLT) (2005). The rates are much higher for groups with other pre-existing conditions such as Down syndrome. The burden on carers is a well-recognised phenomenon. Ramig et al. (2001) give prevalence figures for PD in the USA of 1,000 in every 100,000 (i.e. 1:100) over the age of 60, and Duffy (2005) gives an estimate of dysarthria in 60% of the PD population. The movement disorder in PD affects communication in a number of ways, most obviously as dysarthria, but also in various nonverbal aspects of communication.

Given the variety in types of dementia and variability in progression of the condition, it is difficult to summarise the likely speech and language therapy role, though it is generally considered to be wide-ranging. According to the RCSLT Position Paper (2005), the role includes direct work with clients and involvement with carers and other professionals with a view to enabling people 'to retain a sense of independence/self-worth and remain at home for as long as possible' (p. 8). The issues associated with this broad role provide some of the material for Scenario 7.1.

The traditional speech and language therapy role in PD has generally had a more established focus on direct therapy aimed at remediation of the motor speech disorder and associated communication skills. In many parts of the world the last decade has seen one particular approach to intervention in PD dysarthria – the Lee Silvermann Voice Treatment® (see Sapir, Ramig & Fox, 2006, for an overview) – promoted as a 'gold standard'. It is this approach that forms the backdrop to Scenario 7.2.

This chapter does not include one aspect of degenerative conditions that is widely discussed in medical ethics textbooks, namely terminal care (Scenario 3.2, p. 43). Although SLTs are involved with people in the final stages of progressive disease, a good example being motor neurone disease, the availability of discussion in other texts suggested that we might alternatively turn our attention to some of the ostensibly less dramatic aspects of the earlier stages of the conditions which are not addressed elsewhere.

Scenario 7.1

In Scenario 7.1 in this chapter we focus on a domiciliary service for people with dementia. Sophie, a student SLT, is on her way to a home visit in the company of Rita, a volunteer with a community group. They are going to see Elsie, who has dementia, and her husband, Harold. Sophie is pondering both the forthcoming visit and her own forthcoming placement report.

Two buckets, some cloths, rubber gloves and a small collection of cleaning products. It made a change from language assessment materials. No sign of any lightbulbs, though.

'I don't really feel very comfortable with this idea,' said Sophie, turning round to face the front of the car again.

'Possibly not, Sophie, but then if you want to feel comfortable, you should stay in bed. We don't come to work to be comfortable; we come to work to help people live their lives to their full potential.'

Student is inflexible and has difficulty thinking about wider issues.

Was there a category for that on the form? Sophie was due to sit down with her speech and language therapy supervisor at the end of the week to complete the clinical placement report and she wasn't quite sure how much influence Rita Bleasdale had on this process. Rita appeared to have rather a lot of influence on rather a lot of processes. She'd been around for ever and knew all the staff.

Sophie thought the six-week placement had gone fairly well and she had enjoyed working with Nadia, the SLT with overall responsibility for the placement. But these community visits with Rita had been a challenge from day one. Rita was a volunteer with Community Voluntary Action and she was a woman who Got Things Done. She had been assigned to Harold and Elsie to help with domestic activities and they, like most of the families she worked with, seemed to view her as some sort of unofficial family member. Nadia had been very keen for Sophie to learn about the 'statutory service – voluntary agency interface'. Which was Rita. 'We'd be lost without that service,' Nadia had told her. Sophie couldn't help wondering where therapy was supposed to fit in all this.

Rita and Sophie were in Rita's car on their way to see Mr and Mrs York. Harold and Elsie. Most of the shops on the street were boarded up. There was a patch of open ground in front of where Harold and Elsie lived and some kids were chasing a dog across it. 'I don't suppose it looks much like this where you live, does it Sophie?' This topic had come up several times when they were driving to and from appointments but Rita never seemed to tire of it. 'You have to think differently here because people's lives are different to what you're used to.'

Student needs to pay greater attention to the whole client.

Last week they had had another awkward conversation on the way back from the appointment when Sophie had questioned whether it was really in their best interests for Harold and Elsie to stay living in their own home. Elsie seemed much more disorientated than she had been four weeks ago and the dementia was making her do some very strange things. Harold had evidently recovered quite a bit from his second stroke, but he hardly seemed in a fit state to look after himself, let alone Elsie.

'What do you think will happen if Elsie has to leave?' Rita had asked, forcefully. 'She'll get even more confused in a home and she'll deteriorate even faster than she is doing at the moment. What we can do while she's at home is to support her version of reality so that she doesn't get too distressed. She's convinced that her son is still alive and is just out at work. Even though she gets confused about it, there's no way she's going to accept that he isn't. If she goes into a good home, they'll insist on trying to reorientate her to reality; if she goes into a bad one, who knows what will happen. I've known them ever since Harold's first stroke. They only have each other. If you separate them, they won't last six months.'

That sounded fine in theory, but as far as Sophie could see, relationships with the neighbours were deteriorating rapidly. Harold said if he didn't watch her carefully she was out of the door and banging on whichever door took her fancy. Mostly she just asked when Jim was coming home because his meal was getting cold, but increasingly she would shout at whoever came to the door. Reactions were starting to polarise. Some people still led Elsie gently back home. Others just shouted back that she was mad and ought to be locked up.

Harold was always pleased to see Rita and she pretty much had the run of the place. The previous week Rita had picked Harold's wallet up from the table and taken some money, telling Sophie she needed to buy them some spare lightbulbs and she'd bring them with her next time. Sophie had tried looking surreptitiously round the car but she couldn't see them. It seemed a bit rude to ask Rita directly.

This was a big day for Harold and Elsie. The people from the Social Work department were coming round to assess their situation and make a decision about whether they could stay living as they were. Rita had insisted on being present. The other thing that Rita had insisted on was going an hour early so they could help Harold get the place cleaned up before the assessment visit.

Rita took up the baton again. 'It's all very well bandying around terms like multi-disciplinary, but not everything in people's lives fits neatly into a pigeonhole. What's supposed to happen about the things that nobody claims responsibility for? If the social workers start to think Harold and Elsie can't manage by themselves, they'll have Elsie in a home quicker than you can rinse out a mop. So we're just going to lend a little helping hand, whether you feel comfortable with it or not, Sophie.'

Another phrase destined for the report loomed in front of Sophie's eyes:

Student is reluctant to get her hands dirty.

Commentary on Scenario 7.1

Claire Penn

We have in this scenario an impaired elderly couple living in constrained circumstances who have restricted decision-making capacity. Yet a decision must be made about their future. They are clearly vulnerable – Elsie because of a dementing condition and Harold because of two strokes. How this decision is to be made presents a huge challenge to family, carers and professionals.

Harold and Elsie are not the only vulnerable persons here. Sophie is feeling very vulnerable. Unlike much of the SLT's caseload, the harsh reality of this type of client is deterioration and decline. Such reality is particularly hard for the student SLT. What if these were my grandparents? What would I want in this situation?

The interface with other professionals and with other lay care workers such as Rita is a common feature of such community care. 'Teamwork' is a splendid textbook term which assumes a profoundly different meaning in the reality of context. How can we as professionals, whose role in the team may be new or even transient, be heard and be trusted? How can Sophie, as a young outsider, first understand and then, importantly, influence positively this set of circumstances? This, after all, is her perceived duty – why she was called to the profession. She is feeling powerless and inadequate.

There are three main components to this complex puzzle: the environment, the participants and the actions. The environment seems no longer conducive to supporting the aim of doing good and minimizing harm for Elsie and Harold. The shops are boarded up, the neighbours apparently unreliable. Clearly there are no safeguards which prevent Elsie from wandering. Harold seems to bear an unreasonable burden of responsibility. Yet the environment clearly provides a familiarity and a security for this old couple. A change of environment has the potential (real or imagined) to hasten the degeneration.

The participants are of interest. We conjecture that Elsie is in the moderate stages of dementia. Harold, although he appears still able to communicate, has had two strokes and it is therefore likely that his mobility has been affected. He is certainly unlikely to be able to manage with the daily demands of cleaning, washing, shopping and cooking as well as caring for his wife's safety and nutrition. We assume this is why a volunteer has been appointed. The role and the power of this volunteer are unclear in this scenario. We know little of the nursing service and Rita appears to have assumed a role which for Sophie is unexpected.

Sophie is clearly very aware of her status as student. She has a fear of evaluation (possibly framed by some previous negative experiences). She has a lack of confidence in her ability to make judgements. She is feeling uncomfortable about some of the things that she has seen. She is worried about Rita's judgement and she suspects that Rita's interest in this couple extends beyond their safety and comfort. Sophie feels unsafe about expressing these concerns, is bewildered about the relevance of her role in this community placement and unfortunately seems to be lacking appropriate supervision. Above all, Sophie is a person. Regardless of her youth and her stage of training, she is responding to a human condition in a human way. She has hunches and intuitions and a set of moral standards which make this scenario uncomfortable for her. She may not have read the ethics textbooks yet, but of course she knows right from wrong. And she is feeling ethical distress. She needs to learn to formulate what about this situation is making her feel uncomfortable. Ethics will provide her with the tools and the vocabulary to do this and can guide her into steps which will make her feel more powerful.

Sophie has a right to regular meetings with her supervisor, Nadia, and should feel encouraged without fear of evaluation to voice some of her concerns. Nadia must in this case be willing and able to function as a wise and virtuous role-model and facilitate the process of ethical problem solving by helping Sophie identify why this is an ethical problem, and guiding her to move forward mindfully.

For example, Nadia might suggest the following framework of ethical problem solving:

░ Gather as much information as possible.
░ Consider available options and their outcomes
░ Whose interests are served by these options?
░ What are the steps required?
░ Who should implement these steps?

We need more information here to help the process. We do not know what criteria are applied by Social Work in making a decision about moving the elderly couple, but we sincerely hope that such criteria are transparent and that they do not depend (as Rita would imply) solely on the cleanliness of the environment. It is necessary that Sophie finds out what the criteria are.

There should be an assessment of decision-making capacity. Has anyone asked Harold what he wants? If he has difficulty communicating, Sophie's role becomes particularly critical. Elsie's preferences might also be discernible through suitable scaffolded communication techniques.

We do not know enough about the options of placement. Rita implies that the couple will be separated. This is clearly an undesirable and inhumane option, but is it reality? What are the cost and availability of such options? What facilities exist and how are couples managed in such facilities? How is the transition managed? What does research tell us about the impact of such transition?

What is the legal and financial status of the couple? Have advance directives been made? If Harold is still controlling the finances, what safeguards are in place to ensure he is being supported?

We know there is one son who has died, but are there other family members who can be involved in the decision? If so, how can they be traced?

If there is a team, who else is on it and what do they think? Other professionals' opinions are clearly important here. We might be interested, for example, in the opinions of an occupational therapist, a dietician and a neuropsychologist.

The possible options of placement will unfortunately depend on the context in which they are being made. Economic aspects frame the choices in many countries. However, within such constraints the consequences of each option (e.g. preserving status quo, modifying status quo and increasing support, moving Elsie alone to suitable care or moving the couple to suitable care) should be imagined both in the short term and in the long term.

There should be a risk and benefit analysis, and no step should be taken before there is a careful team decision which is made through such an analysis. The goal should be to maximize good and minimize harm. The team in this case should include the clients themselves, the professionals and of course the volunteer. Whose interest will these decisions serve? Sophie must also think of consequences for herself in helping resolve this problem. Perhaps the most important consequence can be framed by the following question: 'How will this make me feel?' (or 'How will I sleep at night?').

Once the team decision has been made, there is someone who should implement that step. If the move is recommended, the Social Work team is likely to be supervising the move, but other team members will need to be involved. Continuity of care is critical, and quality of care and quality of life, though related, are certainly different constructs.

What on earth does speech and language therapy have to do with all this, thinks Sophie? Sophie's role is critically important in facilitating and enabling communication with the team. She can develop a relationship with Elsie and Harold; she can be the researcher, the observer and the facilitator. She can certainly help establish decision-making capacity and aid the expression, understanding and appreciation of choice. She can systematically gather information about the options and their potential outcomes. She has a right to expect support from her supervisor during this process, so she can move from ethical distress via a process of systematic reflection towards a position of increased confidence in her role as a useful and effective moral agent. There is, in my opinion, no better context for that professional journey than the field of dementia.

Claire Penn, Professor and Chair, Department of Speech Pathology and Audiology, University of the Witwatersrand, South Africa

Commentary on Scenario 7.1

Travis T. Threats

The road to hell is paved with good intentions.

This case involves the ethical conduct of a volunteer, Rita, who a speech-language pathology student, Sophie, has been assigned to as part of her overall learning experience. There are several ethical concerns addressed in this scenario. One area of concern is the ethical responsibilities of volunteers. Another area is the conduct of the student being put into this situation. And a third area is the ethical responsibilities of the service organization and the university.

Volunteers could be reasonably expected to follow similar ethics as professionals working in fields such as speech-language pathology, where being licensed and being able to practice in the profession can be jeopardized by being judged to have behaved in an unethical manner. Volunteers might also reasonably be expected to act within the same ethical guidelines as the organizations that utilize them. In that sense, they are subject to many, though not all, of the guidelines for professionals in that organization. Organizations that use volunteers would be wise to provide them with training and discussion of ethics. Discussions of crossing boundaries – including the sense of entitlement that someone is 'your' patient – would be a regular part of this training. Volunteers who work with the elderly should be cautioned that the population served is vulnerable and thus easily swayed by their opinions. It is also not unusual for organizations to make volunteers sign a written agreement that they will adhere to certain ethical standards.

In this case, we have a volunteer fighting the good cause, openly cutting corners in order to do what she considers right, even though she should be able to tell from the reaction and questions of the student that all does not seem right. Rita is essentially arguing that whatever boundaries may be crossed, it is worth it. In other words, morality dictates that we sometimes go beyond the rules of the situation. Is it right, for example, to deceive if a greater good is achieved?

But in this case, whose needs are being serviced? Are the couple's needs being met or are the needs of Rita's ego being met? Sophie has heard reports of the client wandering around the neighborhood and some of the neighbors being openly hostile, and of the husband's questionable health. If Elsie ends up physically harmed during her wandering, would Rita still feel that she had 'protected' the couple? Perhaps the husband would indeed like more help in at least an assistive living or possibly a nursing home environment, but Rita could be talking him out of it.

According to Rita, other professionals do not have the couple's best interest in mind. She can make the house look better than it is, to fool the social worker, and it seems that she stays during the visit to make sure to intercept the social workers' concerns and counter them. She is openly disparaging of other health professionals to Sophie, which itself violates expected ethical behavior as a volunteer in that it questions the actions of others without proof – just as wrong as making *a priori* judgments about persons of a given race or socioeconomic level. On that same note, her pejorative remarks about Sophie's supposedly privileged background also are prejudicial and thus have no place in any clinical or helping environment. If a student has questions about the wisdom or safety of an approach, the way for Rita to deal with them is to openly discuss the concerns and not attack the student for asking, unless, of course, she feels that she has something to hide. In the ethical guidelines for many organizations, workers and volunteers alike are encouraged to discuss openly any possible ethical dilemmas.

Up to this point the assumption has been that this is a case of good intentions carried to the extreme. But Sophie's statement that Rita is almost a family member and is taking money directly from someone's wallet means that it is possible that more than ethical boundaries are being crossed here. Rita's behavior may in fact be criminal. If any of the money is for Rita's personal use, it *is* criminal. If Rita is blocking information from the couple about possible government benefits to elevate their 'need' of her, this would be highly unethical, and possibly also criminal if used for personal financial gain by Rita. Sophie has seen only *this* blatant unethical behavior, but what about other possible scams such as cashing checks for them, having them put her on power of attorney, or putting her name on bank accounts or insurance? Maybe Rita only made up the questionable lightbulb story because Sophie saw her take the money. Volunteers are not liable in a professional sense, but they are considered liable personally. That is, the government, the clients or the organization that uses them can sue the person for any harm that may come from their actions. They can also be found criminally negligent, as even a member of a person's own family could.

There are also ethical concerns for the university and for Sophie. Does the university or Sophie's academic department know the situation that she is in? They may be putting Sophie at risk for future ability to receive a license if she is shown to be complicit in what she knew was unethical or even illegal behavior. The agency and school seem to think the world of Rita who has been assigned to oversee this experience for Sophie. How deeply have they looked into what she does? The department may have failed its professional ethical responsibility to put students in sites with persons who can model all aspects of professional behavior. If the agency has had any complaints, these should be relayed to the academic departments to allow them to make the decision as to whether to place students there.

Finally, Sophie herself is in a precarious ethical situation. In movies, the hero stands up to an injustice against the odds, takes a few licks and in the end is vindicated and recognized by all as a hero. In real life, people stand up to an injustice or ethically dubious behavior by their superiors and they may lose – get bad evaluations, get fired and sometimes get overtly discredited. Ethical behavior is not the easiest road. Sophie is very concerned about what she has seen but is equally concerned that speaking out will lower her grade. Considering the positive comments everyone in authority over her has made about Rita, she justly fears that speaking out will elicit exactly the comments she imagines will be written in her evaluation. She can stay quiet and lose a little of her soul or speak up and possibly lose a lot of her grade. Sophie should talk frankly, with specific examples, to her supervisor, Nadia, about the situation. Sophie could then gauge the response of her supervisor. Nadia might react by putting her head in the sand, or by attacking – or at least questioning – Sophie's right to impugn her past judgment. If Sophie questions Rita's behavior, she may put herself in a difficult position. If Sophie tells her supervisor what has happened, in this case she has done the ethically correct thing and notified those in authority about her concerns. And yes, it is even possible that she could be graded down because of her views. What if the situation seems ethically wrong to Sophie and her academic department refuses to address it? Strictly speaking, she has done her professional ethical duty to report any suspicious activity. If nothing is done by the department and she is graded down for reporting her concerns, then she has demonstrated ethical behavior despite the negative consequences for her.

There is a cold practical reason that Sophie should officially make her feelings known. In case Rita does get publicly exposed as behaving unethically or possibly committing illegal acts, everyone involved could be hurt, including the departments that placed students there. If Sophie is on record, she does not get pulled into the muck because she did all she could do with the power (and evidence) she had. Of course, if she were to put her concerns in writing to the department, it may force the department to withdraw students from the placement even if they do not agree with Sophie, in order to avoid possible future lawsuits themselves. Thus, not only is the road to hell paved with good intentions, but the road to good is sometimes paved with dubious intentions.

Travis T. Threats, Professor and Chair, Department of Communication Sciences and Disorders, Saint Louis University, USA

Scenario 7.2

For Scenario 7.2 we turn our attention from dementia to Parkinson's disease and specifically to Keith Gillespie, who has recently been diagnosed with the condition. The scenario is in the form of two sets of e-mails. The first is between Keith and his son, David. The second is between Keith's SLT, Chinwe Ogunsolu, and her friend from their recent student days, Katy.

From: keith.gillespie@global.net

To: david.gillespie007@global.net

Date: 25 May 2008 11.15

Subject: Getting to grips with technology

Dear David

You've been on at me for ages to drag myself into the 21st century so now seems as good a time as any, especially as even I cannot read my handwriting these days. It's a shame really, I used to enjoy writing. Since it could take me all day at the rate I type, I'll just send this to make sure we are connected.

If you don't receive this, let me know.

Your adventurous father

From: david.gillespie007@global.net

To: keith.gillespie@global.net

Date: 25 May 2008 20.58

Subject: Getting to grips with technology

Dad

At last. Well done, though you might want to run the joke checker over the next one. That's a joke. There's no such thing, though I could make loadsa money if i invented one.

How d'you get on with the speech therapist? Mum said your opinion was that you can 'talk perfectly fine, thank you' and it would be a waste of time. (I'm inclined to agree with you, if I'm honest.) Better go cos J's woken up and I'm on babysitting duty this evening.
David

From: chinwe.ogunsolu@tlv.com

To: KayTee26@webmail.com

Date: 25 May 2008 21.36

Subject: Greetings from The Back Of Beyond

Hello Katy

How's it going in The Big City? Are you still doing all that cultural stuff or has the first flush worn off now that you're in financial meltdown?

Thankfully today has involved less driving and less farm animals than usual cos I've had a day at the clinic for people who're near enough to get to me. Mind you, I wouldn't want to spend all day cooped up in an office.

Here's one we never discussed at college. I had this man referred a while ago with Parkinson's disease – he's not long been diagnosed. Saw him a couple of weeks ago – speech isn't too bad at the moment. He couldn't see the point of speech and language therapy though he agreed to come back today (maybe cos I was nice to him). He refused point blank to meet any other people with PD. Anyway, to cut a long story short, I *happened* to arrange an appointment today that *happened* to overlap with another man with PD, whose speech is really really bad, and *happened* to leave them together in the waiting room for a few minutes and I think it was a bit of a shock for him. Is that a really bad thing to do? Mind you, he's coming back next month so maybe I got the message across. The only problem with that is I've never seen anyone with PD before so I'll have to do some speed-reading...

Say hello to anyone else from college you bump into and tell them if they want some fresh air they know where I am.

Regards

Chinwe

From: KayTee26@webmail.com

To: chinwe.ogunsolu@tlv.com

Date: 27 May 2008 22.05

Subject: Greetings from TBC

Hiya Chinwe

I'm definitely heading for financial meltdown – may have to keep this short to save on electricity! Where's the problem? You worry about things too much. The way I see it, you got an effective job done. They could have met up by chance anyway and now you'll be able to do a proper job. Am really getting into autism now and actually managed a bit of reading the other day. Can't remember any of it, mind. Saw Teresa today – she says hi.

Luv KT

From: keith.gillespie@global.net

To: david.gillespie007@global.net

Date: 28 May 2008 14.35

Subject: The perils of speech therapy

Dear David

Quite exciting getting e-mails, though not the same as a proper letter with a proper stamp. You're quite right, I didn't see the point of speech therapy and I'm not really sure I do now. I only went because your mother says she can't understand anything I say but then she's been saying that for years. It must be her hearing. I met another man at the clinic with PD whose speech was awful, so that's worried me a bit. I thought it was suspicious that his appointment was so close to mine but Chinwe (that's the therapist) didn't admit to anything. She's very friendly. She's given me three appointments over the next two months to do something or other so I'll keep you informed.

The drugs are a bit unpredictable. Some days I feel really good and then other times I get stuck in door frames. No, I haven't put on that much weight – I just can't get through them. Your mother has to distract me by talking about something else before I can move. Really embarrassing (having your mother talk to me in public – ha ha!).

Talking of your mother, she has a big space on the calendar in July. I'm sure it's about the right size for writing 'David/Connie/Jessica visiting'. Thought I'd better warn you ...

CyberDad

From: david.gillespie007@global.net

To: keith.gillespie@global.net

Date: 10 June 2008 07.10

Subject: Speech

Dad

Sorry it's taken a while to get back to you. Job, baby, wife, house etc.

Was browsing the net last night and did a search for you on PD and speech stuff. Came up with some details of therapy that sounds like it's been really effective for other people. Says it has to be done intensively or not at all. That doesn't sound like what you're getting so you should ask the therapist.

I'll send you the link.

Gotta go to work. See you in July.

D

From: chinwe.ogunsolu@tlv.com

To: KayTee26@webmail.com

Date: 1 July 2008 16.58

Subject: help!

Hello again Katy

Lots of animals today. I'm starting to recognise individual sheep, which is a bit worrying. It's a miracle the car's still holding out considering the distances I'm doing.

The man I told you about with PD – I've seen him a couple of times and we've done some Lee Silverman-type stuff. Then this afternoon I got a call from his son, who was – how shall I put it – quite assertive. He says he's been searching the net for info on PD and he came across all this evidence that speech work has to be done intensively to be effective and that means n times a week for n number of weeks and that doesn't sound like what his dad's getting. It's definitely not what his dad's getting. The chances of his dad getting intensive therapy out here are about as remote as my house is. I suppose I could see if he wants to go to some 'specialist', wherever that might be. I told him we were working on a programme that was adapted to suit the circumstances. It was the best I could come up with under pressure.

Help!

Chinwe

Commentary on Scenario 7.2

Deborah Theodoros

This scenario provides a realistic insight into a common situation encountered by clients with PD in rural areas. The case highlights several important ethical issues relating to the management of communication disorders in progressive conditions, growing health consumerism, professional development, evidenced-based practice, and service delivery in rural areas.

PD evokes ethical dilemmas and challenges for SLTs as a result of the slow and insidious rate of progression of the disease, the highly variable presentation of symptoms, and the differential impact of the disease on quality of life. For some people with PD, changes in speech and voice will have a dramatic impact on their capacity to function in social and vocational roles, while for others, these symptoms may be less disconcerting. The case presented in this scenario clearly demonstrates the early signs of deterioration in speech and voice which at this stage are not considered by the client to be problematic. Keith's apparent lack of awareness of the changes in his speech is a common feature of many people with PD in the early stages of the disease and is thought to be due to an inherent sensory dysfunction. It is well known, however, that Keith's speech and voice production will deteriorate over time and, slowly but surely, impact on his quality of life. The initial challenge for Chinwe, the SLT in this scenario, is to determine how best to provide education to Keith about the inevitable effects of PD on speech in an appropriate and sensitive manner to enable him to make an informed decision about treatment. A further dilemma arises for Chinwe in determining the optimal course of management for

Keith within her scope of practice in a rural setting. While early intervention at this point in time is important in order to delay the progressive effects of the disease on speech and maintain functional communication, she is faced with the reality that such treatment cannot be provided at the required level due to caseload priorities and restricted access to the client.

This scenario also highlights a more recent challenge for SLTs, namely growing health consumerism. SLTs need to be prepared to meet the demands of the growing health consumerism in today's society where individuals and their families are becoming increasingly proactive in their healthcare. With expanding access to information on the internet, more and more people seek information about their conditions and treatment alternatives from a multitude of websites and electronic resources. Keith's son, David, has researched his father's condition, and in this scenario is probably more informed than the SLT about treatment options. In this case, consumer knowledge has presented a challenge to Chinwe, who is ill-prepared to discuss the nature of the speech disorder and treatment options with a family member. As a result, Chinwe faces considerable pressure from Keith's son, who expects that optimal treatment will be provided to his father regardless of location. Chinwe's apparent lack of initiative in updating her current knowledge of PD and treatment options reflects a low commitment to ongoing professional development. Such behaviour will inevitably result in ongoing conflict and challenges for her in her clinical practice.

As a result of her inadequate knowledge base, Chinwe did not meet her professional responsibility to employ evidence-based practice in this case. Her failure to recognise the importance of administering a proven efficacious treatment to Keith in the manner required could be considered professionally unethical. While the inherent difficulties of rural practice are acknowledged, they should not detract from either providing the most effective treatment available to a client or seeking an alternative way in which this could be achieved.

The clinical setting of this scenario exemplifies the professional and service delivery issues faced by rural and remote practitioners. Not only does Chinwe experience professional isolation, but the tyranny of distance impacts significantly on the quality and efficiency of her service delivery. Her need to drive long distances to see a client on an infrequent basis would seem to negate the effects of any treatment provided. The challenge for Chinwe is to determine ways in which her therapy can be delivered in a time-effective manner without compromising quality of care.

The management of this case was fraught with several ethical issues and challenges which were either not recognised by Chinwe or ineffectively managed. Her initial attempt to educate Keith about his speech problem failed unequivocally, with her client no more informed about his condition, and, if anything, made to feel anxious about his future. Counselling clients with progressive disorders should be handled with the utmost sensitivity so as not to engender unnecessary concern in the client. Information regarding the effects of PD on speech should be provided, questions answered, and the client and family given the opportunity to reflect on this information, and request additional input as required. In this case Chinwe should have adopted a transparent and positive approach to delivering such information to Keith, in order to avoid misconceptions and concerns. In her ill-conceived attempt to inform Keith about the effects of PD on speech, she failed to provide sufficient information for him to understand his need for treatment at this stage of his disease. Furthermore, where it is the case that the most effective treatment cannot be provided in a particular setting, the client's understanding of the speech problem and treatment options is crucial in the decision to seek treatment elsewhere. With her lack of in-depth knowledge of her client's communication disorder, treatment options, and the importance of adhering to the principles of evidence-based practice, Chinwe's management of her client is virtually ineffectual and should be discontinued in its present form. Chinwe needs to seek advice from an experienced clinician working in the area of PD to determine an alternative management plan for her client. In this particular rural setting, it is possible that Keith and his family may need to consider moving temporarily to an area where he could receive the most efficacious treatment (Lee Silverman Voice Treatment [LSVT®]) (Ramig et al., 2001).

Professionally, Chinwe needs to initiate an ongoing development program including external and self-generated continuing education, as well as mentoring with a senior SLT to ensure that her knowledge is continually updated. In view of her rural setting and the physical logistics of her practice it is imperative that Chinwe reassess her methods of service delivery, exploring other models that may be used to supplement or replace face-to-face treatment. Alternatives such as computer-based therapy activities and telehealth applications involving videoconferencing might be considered feasible for some clients.

With degenerative conditions expected to increase with the ageing population worldwide, and the health budget continuing to decline, SLTs are destined to meet perplexing challenges in addressing the communication needs of this population. As demonstrated in this scenario, ethical issues that arise will require SLTs to be innovative, responsive to changing social trends, and academically and professionally prepared.

Deborah Theodoros, Professor and Head, Division of Speech Pathology & Co-Director, Telerehabilitation Research Unit, University of Queensland, Australia

Commentary on Scenario 7.2

Kartini Ahmad

The scenario portrayed here is familiar in Malaysia, where speech pathology services (and many other specialized health and allied health services) are relatively newly developed and not yet fully established in many disciplines. A young clinician may be running a one-person show in a small health district and seeing all kinds of people who appear at the door. Clinicians may not have experience of a particular disorder but they have to see and manage the patient nevertheless; otherwise the only option is to refer the patient to a specialized center in the major cities – most likely beyond reach of many ordinary patients. Situations like this happen because, unlike their medical counterparts, the speech pathology profession in this country does not yet impose a period of internship or apprenticeship for new graduates, mainly due to the relative lack of experienced professionals to provide the training. To complicate matters, sometimes newly qualified clinicians could be posted to less popular districts, more often in rural or remote areas, whereas more experienced clinicians would move on to a more senior position in the larger or more urban setup.

Ideally a clinician should be equipped with the knowledge and skills to see and manage any patient in the clinic. It is only fair that the patient gets the best possible treatment from a well-trained, experienced and informed clinician. The reality, however, is far from the ideal and it happens everywhere and in many disciplines, not confined to speech pathology alone. In the real job situation a clinician may be forced to take on cases for which he/she may have very little experience. For example, not everyone will have had experience working with a laryngectomee during their training. Others may not have seen the more rare cases of voice disorder because of the limited cases in the voice clinic during their clinical block. Newly qualified clinicians can be understandably anxious and feel ill equipped when faced with such situations, but they should know that no school or college could possibly equip students with all the necessary skills and knowledge upon graduation. People learn many new things only after they have started working, and they do this from peers, mentors and from their own reading. In fact many new frontiers are opened via chance discovery and self-learning.

In the situation described above the dilemma is whether to turn the patient away or to treat the patient with 'sub-optimal' treatment. Neither option is ideal but the second option may be considered on condition the clinician goes on to find out as much information as she can about the treatment before the next appointment. Most times the clinician will already have some idea about the line of management but may not have the exact details of the techniques. Sometimes even knowing the details of the technique may not be adequate until they are being applied and practised with the patient. Therefore unless the clinician is doing something far removed from the norms for the treatment of such conditions, she is not practising unethically. Of course this should not be taken as a blanket rule that applies to all cases, but should be limited only to non-life-threatening cases. A caveat must be placed for cases requiring instrumentation or specific procedures involving airway, such as videofluoroscopy and laryngeal endoscopy, where experience is absolutely required.

Another dilemma is whether to practise the Lee Silverman technique as prescribed or to modify the technique to suit the patient's needs and/or the clinician's level of skill. Lee Silverman is a highly prescribed technique, and unless one is a certified Lee Silverman practitioner one cannot claim to be using the technique. In that sense the issue is straightforward. However, the Lee Silverman technique also derives its principles from many other techniques used before it and the clinician may avoid the controversies and take a safe route by not claiming that she is using a particular technique but instead explaining to the patient the principles of the management that she will be working on for the period.

A further dilemma in the case scenario is whether it is ethical for a clinician to deliberately arrange a meeting between patients. In the case above the meeting was unsolicited and instinctively the clinician herself appears to have some doubts about its acceptability, hence the assurance she seeks from her colleague in the e-mail. It is quite presumptuous of her to assume her patient would appreciate the meeting or that they could have met by chance anyway. The patient was so uncomfortable afterwards that he mentioned it to his son in the e-mail. He also felt suspicious about the 'chance meeting' and asked the clinician directly about it. Even though she denied it, he was not convinced by her denial and so an unnecessary mistrust has been sown from the start of the relationship. Perhaps some kind of permission could have been sought first before arranging the meeting.

Possibly another minor ethical issue here is whether clinicians should divulge information about patients to friends and colleagues through e-mail conversations under the guise of consultation. To me, as long as personal identification is respected I would let this issue rest. In modern times like the present, e-mails have replaced phone and face-to-face conversation and it is an excellent way to get connected for consultation with colleagues and peers. It is more so in remote areas where clinicians might practise in isolation. In the case above, however, the e-mail was not really for consultation as the colleague was also not experienced in the area; her area seemed to be in autism. So it is debatable whether the e-mail exchange is a consultative e-mail or just a casual one, although the possible benefits of checking actions with our peers are important.

In the Malaysian context, divulging patient information to close relatives or family members may be seen quite differently depending on the setting. In many rural families here in Malaysia, patient management may require consensus from elder family members or the head of the family, regardless of age. It may not be the patient's decision to undergo treatment but may involve relatives calling family members for a meeting and divulging important information regarding the patient. In more urbanized societies this may be seen as an absolute breach of a patient's confidentiality but may be an acceptable practice in some areas elsewhere. In situations like this the clinician needs to understand and balance professional practice and local practice and the boundaries surrounding each.

Kartini Ahmad, Associate Professor, Head of Department of Audiology and Speech Sciences, Faculty of Allied Health Sciences, Universiti Kebangsaan Malaysia

Discussion

The challenges that SLTs are destined to meet in their work with people with PD are described by Theodoros as 'perplexing', and the same can safely be said of work in dementia. In this section we discuss the challenges of telling the truth, of how to act in the presence of potentially unethical behaviour (especially if you are a student) and whether ethical standards are – or can be – the same in remote rural practice and newly developing services as they are in more highly resourced contexts and established services. Finally, we look at some of the challenges of maintaining confidentiality.

In Scenario 7.2 Chinwe has a responsibility to educate Mr Gillespie about the course of PD and what he can expect to encounter. He needs the information to be able to make informed, autonomous decisions about how he deals with the development of the condition. The commentators agree that Chinwe's chosen method for alerting Mr Gillespie to future difficulties with speech – by covertly arranging for him to meet someone whose speech he perceives as 'awful' – is at best clumsy and at worst insensitive and ill-conceived. Even if she has his best interests at heart, the net result is a greater increase in his anxiety than in his level of knowledge or understanding and, as Ahmad says, this also sows the seeds of an unnecessary mistrust.

Telling the truth

This is not to say, of course, that Chinwe's task is easy. Theodoros refers to the need for a transparent and positive approach to delivering information in a situation where Mr Gillespie does not yet perceive there to be a problem (or attributes it to his wife's hearing). The problem that Chinwe faces is, in essence, about the complexities of telling patients the truth. Mr Gillespie's speech will inevitably deteriorate. Chinwe knows this. Mr Gillespie doesn't, but by some means or other he needs to, in order to understand the role of therapy and whether or not to engage with it. The notion of telling the truth is discussed widely in texts on healthcare ethics (e.g. Beauchamp & Childress, 2009; A. Campbell, Gillett & Jones 2001). Despite being generally regarded as central to good relationships between professionals and patients, there is also recognition that truthfulness is by no means a unitary or straightforward concept. For example, what *is* the truth here? How much will Mr Gillespie's speech deteriorate? How quickly? And crucially, how much does he need to know *now?* Clinicians frequently have to navigate the dividing line between different interpretations of truth in any particular situation.

There is no absolute standard by which the truth can be measured. For example, in this context it could range anywhere from a broad description of PD as a degenerative condition to a detailed account of the biochemical processes involved at synaptic junctions and predicted changes in these processes over time. Mr Gillespie himself has a significant influence on the 'truth', in terms both of the likely progression of his motor speech disorder, given all the other factors relating to him as an individual, and (as also highlighted below in relation to Scenario 7.1) of his perceived receptiveness to information. As Sim (1997) points out, what patients are likely to need is not necessarily *all* the information (whatever that may be) but *sufficient* information to make whatever choices are relevant to them at this point in their lives.

One factor that may underlie Chinwe's actions is what Beauchamp and Childress (2009) refer to as truth dumping, where clinicians divest themselves of potentially painful information quickly, in the name of telling the truth. We might usefully refer back at this point to the example described in Chapter 1 involving Mrs Davies and the seemingly innocuous word 'yet' as another case of an understandable but ultimately damaging therapeutic action. Beauchamp and Childress also discuss the concept of staged disclosure, i.e. giving information at a rate that is perceived to match patients' desire to know and capacity to assimilate the implications. Giving someone information to the effect that they are going to experience an inevitable decrease in function is an intrinsically delicate and ethically sensitive process. On the other hand, Mr Gillespie cannot make informed decisions without reliable information, and if Chinwe can manage a positive, supportive and possibly gradual approach to this interaction, she can potentially save him from the unfettered and aimless anxiety that he might otherwise feel. For Chinwe, as a newly qualified clinician, this is a significant challenge and one for which she seeks support from her friend. A more formal mentoring relationship with an experienced clinician might provide more appropriately targeted support.

Reality orientation

A further aspect of truth-telling arises in Scenario 7.1 in relation to Elsie's version of reality, in which her son is still alive and will shortly be returning home from work. Rita's view is that Elsie should be allowed – and possibly facilitated – to continue in her belief and that any form of reality orientation is simply going to cause her avoidable distress. Sophie is less sure and is concerned that this may be contributing to deteriorating relationships with the neighbours. This divergence of views represents a common problem in dementia care, one that Yang-Lewis and Moody (1995) describe as surfacing on a daily basis, in essence a conflict between orientation to some form of external reality and validation of the patient's reality. In a case study commentary on a similar situation to Rita's ('The Forgetful Mourner', in which nursing home staff ponder the best course of action with Mrs C, a woman with Alzheimer's disease who has forgotten that she attended her son's funeral), Yang-Lewis and Moody individually present very different perspectives on this challenge.

Yang-Lewis proposes that any decision *not* to find some way of conveying that the son has died would require 'a fundamental revision in the staff's perception of Mrs C, from a person with a disease to a person so diseased as to be incapable of comprehending a momentous event in her life' (Yang-Lewis & Moody, 1995, p. 32). He sees anything other than telling this truth as serving to increase the patient's isolation. Moody, on the other hand, compares – in rather startling prose – the nursing and medical staff who make repeated efforts to inform Mrs C that her son has died to 'the torturers of the Spanish Inquisition [who] sincerely believe in the tenets of their faith' and to 'a fanatic who redoubles his efforts having lost sight of the goal' (p. 33). Importantly, he asks whether the patient's *receptivity* to the truth should not be a factor in decisions about how to act.

These two approaches differ fundamentally. Reality orientation views telling the truth (setting aside the difficulty of identifying what constitutes the truth) as a way of keeping the patient connected with reality. Truth-telling is much less important in the validation approach, in which the aim is not to enhance the patient's view of reality but to accept the patient as he or she is (Parker & Dickenson, 2001). This approach was recently highlighted in an article on a dementia unit in the UK *Guardian* newspaper where the manager was quoted as saying. 'We let them live in their own reality and [we] react to that reality' (Benjamin, 2007, p. 7).

At a practical level it needs to be recognised that complex deception is in fact very difficult to maintain. If Rita supports Elsie's version of reality, although Elsie may not suddenly discover the 'truth', the inevitable involvement of more people than Rita makes more likely a potentially uncomfortable mismatch of incoming information for Elsie, possibly a vague sense that various accounts don't quite fit with each other. Another point to take into account in this decision is that it is likely to be easier for family and friends of someone with dementia to make subtle judgements of the implications of a choice one way or another than it is for staff, and that family and friends may modify their approach depending on the information involved, the level of potential distress both for the person with dementia and for other members of the family, and the likely success of the strategy.

Whistleblowing

The position of Sophie, the SLT student in Scenario 7.1, is not to be envied, given her stark choice as described by Threats: 'She can stay quiet and lose a little of her soul or speak up and possibly lose a lot of her grade.' Her discomfort and sense of vulnerability are compounded by what Penn terms 'the harsh reality of this type of client... deterioration and decline', which Penn notes is particularly hard for student SLTs to accommodate to.

Whistleblowing is a term usually applied to uncovering and reporting large-scale misdemeanour with major potential implications all round. Medical research has seen its fair share of such events: the Olivieiri affair in the early 1990s in Toronto serves as example (see Viens & Savulescu, 2004, for a description). This featured a medical researcher in a long, damaging and eventually very public – and no doubt personally painful – fight with a drug manufacturer and hospital and academic organisations. At its heart it involved serious financial conflicts of interest and the wellbeing (and in some cases lives) of patients.

In comparison, Sophie's concerns about Rita's (mis)conduct and her potential adverse influence (over Harold, Elsie and Sophie herself) might seem somewhat tame. But we have to recognise that 'an accusation of ethical misconduct is fraught with serious consequences for all parties' (Pannbacker, 1998, p. 19), and for an inexperienced and inherently vulnerable student, the anxiety provoked by trying to work out what to do for the best is essentially the same as that of the medical researchers, even if the consequences are different. For one thing, whistleblowing seems to have an unfortunate tendency to backfire on the whistleblower. Sophie may hope for a considered and supportive response from her speech and language therapy supervisor – Penn's 'wise and virtuous role-model' – but she cannot necessarily rely on it.

Like all students, Sophie is subject to the power imbalance between her and the people responsible for assessing her performance, and has a realistic concern about her upcoming report. In fact, her role as a student changes the dynamics that might otherwise be in force in such situations. According to Pannbacker (1998), in a rare discussion of whistleblowing centred on speech and language therapy, 'whistleblowing should occur only after intervention has been attempted, such as an attempt to intervene personally and directly with the person(s) at fault' (p. 18). We would not, however, expect Sophie to take direct responsibility for this. Her responsibility, as outlined by Threats, is to report to Nadia. Her status as student should allow her to do this on the basis of suspicion rather than hard evidence. As such, Sophie's actions may be better described as 'reporting through the chain of command' (Pannbacker, 1998, p. 21) than whistleblowing as such (though this terminological nicety may be scant comfort to Sophie in her deliberation). Even so, given Rita's status as 'almost one of the family', Sophie may be concerned that the potential removal of Rita from the scene could serve to make the couple's situation worse rather than better. Ultimately, though, Sophie's obligation to discuss her concerns with Nadia may be fairly clear. Unless she can be certain (which she can't) that ignoring Rita's activities will bring greater benefit to Harold and Elsie (and all subsequent patients with whom Rita is involved), then, as Penn says, Sophie's reasons for joining the profession are the same ones that impel her to raise the issue with Nadia – to attempt to benefit her patients. Of course, Nadia then faces the challenge not only of whether to confront Rita or her managers but also of the complexities of cross-organisational procedures and negotiation. Such is the nature of reporting unethical behaviour.

Ethical goalposts

Returning to Scenario 7.2, one issue looms particularly large: if you can't (for whatever reason) offer what is generally considered to be the best treatment for a condition, is it acceptable to offer a lesser version of it? The gold standard in question here is the LSVT® and is described by Theodoros as the most efficacious treatment (though we studiously avoid any discussion of the clinical case in relation to this claim), to the extent that Mr Gillespie and his family might need to consider temporary relocation in order to avail themselves of the therapy. The question of what to do if this is difficult or impossible to provide arises partly from the scenario itself, in that Chinwe works in a rural practice characterised by remoteness and what Theodoros describes as 'the tyranny of distance'. An alternative interpre-tation, arising from circumstances familiar to the second commentator, is that Chinwe could be working in a country where speech and language therapy ser-vices are only beginning to be developed and where referral to a specialised centre in the major cities is 'most likely beyond reach of many ordinary patients' (Ahmad).

The central issue here is whether the challenges inherent in either remote rural practice or newly developing practice allow for movement of the ethical goalposts. (These are of course not the only circumstances that prompt this question; some of the others, such as parents for whom a child's communication is a low priority, crop up in other chapters.) Attempts to answer the question could potentially take up the rest of the book but, at the risk of being simplistic and in the interests of stimulating thinking on the subject, it is perhaps instructive to consider a difference between ethical and clinical goalposts (though we will dispense with the goalposts metaphor at this point).

It would be difficult to sustain an argument that all health services must have the 'best' clinical system for any particular condition, the implication being that any falling below this standard are somehow behaving unethically. Such an argument applied across the board would render the perception of most healthcare as unethical. We therefore accept wide variation in healthcare resourcing and delivery as being, as it were, a fact of life.

The perspectives taken by the commentators on the delivery of treatment for PD reflect differences in clinical standards underpinned by clinical resources.

An approach such as LSVT® might be the best course of action (until the possible time when some other improvement comes along) *if it is within practical reach*. Theodoros's view of Chinwe's situation is that specialised intervention is sufficiently within reach for her to be faced with the ethical decision as to what is best for Mr Gillespie and what is the best allocation of her resources. It might well be the case that in the circumstances described by Ahmad, a specialised service would not be within practical reach without disastrous knock-on effects for other services and other clients, as a result of which Chinwe does not have the same ethical options. We should also bear in mind the choice of the person potentially receiving the service, in that he may, for a variety of reasons, not feel able to engage with a highly formal and/or intensive therapy programme.

Confidentiality

The political and cultural context within which clinical work takes place can have implications for all areas of practice. This is raised in Scenario 7.2 in relation to the telephone call between Mr Gillespie's son David and Chinwe. Since it is David who has made the call, Chinwe is obliged to have a conversation about David's father, the content of which can range from polite refusal to discuss confidential issues to frank discussion of diagnosis, prognosis, clinical management and Mr Gillespie's emotional state.

According to Hendrick (2000), it is one of the most fundamental aspects of healthcare that patients can expect that information they give health professionals will remain secret. Of course, this is a practical impossibility in the context of any level of either teamworking or family inclusion, and Hendrick also recognises that there is 'little, if any, clear definition of what the term "confidential" means' (p. 92). Discussions within medical ethics tend to focus on the conditions required to make breach of confidentiality permissible, formulated in terms of obligations posed by dangers to third parties (e.g. serious transmissible diseases, threats of violence) and legal requirements to pass on information. Such occasions do arise in speech and language therapy, but once again the focus on relatively dramatic instances serves to obscure the delicate everyday negotiation between patients' rights to set limits on people's access to their lives and the conflicting expectations of healthcare based on teamworking. Teamworking is generally held to include close members of the patient's family, and differing cultural assumptions of family ownership of information serve to complicate this further.

Speech and language therapy codes of ethics invariably include a statement to the effect that SLTs should safeguard clients' confidentiality, though they sometimes offset this with a phrase such as 'unless necessary to protect the welfare of the client or the community' (New Zealand Speech-Language Therapists' Association, 2000, p. 5). Other codes suggest that the SLT should seek a patient's consent to discuss information with other family members, but the nature of that consent is not specified. This view also represents a cultural perspective that may not be in accord with the views of the family involved (as discussed by Ahmad), who may view health information as family property. Indeed, there has been significant work in medical ethics on cultural views of issues such as disclosure of diagnosis (Blackhall, Murphy, Frank, Michel & Azen, 1995; Pucci, Bellardinelli, Borsetti & Giuliani, 2003). The question of who in the healthcare team (or indeed outside it) can reasonably be included in discussion is usually left to a clinician's discretion and often works on the basis of 'unspoken ignorance': most patients simply do not know how many people have been party to discussions about them. As with other subtle, ongoing decision making, written guidelines are unlikely to prove sufficiently sensitive or practical to offer assistance, and individual SLTs have to stay alert in order to balance confidentiality and the patient's best interests.

Summary

It is hardly surprising that progressive conditions give rise to difficult issues, requiring significant adjustments from the person with the condition and the family and a sensitive and empathic approach from professionals. From the moment people are informed of the diagnosis of a degenerative condition, they find themselves on the wrong side of a knowledge gap that needs to be bridged if they are to tackle the future with any confidence. On the other side of the gap is the total of accumulated knowledge about the condition, often personalised in the form of health professionals. Significantly, that accumulated knowledge is also increasingly accessible via support groups and electronic resources, but sometimes the sheer volume of this information can make the learning process more rather than less frightening. The SLT's responsibility is to help such patients bridge the knowledge gap at a manageable pace so that they can maintain as much control over their future as possible.

Where control has moved out of reach, as is the case for Elsie and her husband, the SLT may be faced with very basic questions about the type of approach to use (as in the discussion of reality orientation and validation therapy). As we have seen, perspectives on these approaches can differ fundamentally, and the SLT may need to be alert to daily developments to negotiate a course that suits patient and family. The broad context – political, economic, social – can also influence ethical perspectives on provision of 'gold standard' treatments.

The vulnerability of people in the later stages of progressive conditions means that professionals need to be vigilant for potential abuse, particularly where it comes from people ostensibly in a position to help. In addition, both Scenarios 7.1 and 7.2 involve SLTs with relatively limited experience – one a student, the other newly qualified – whose own vulnerability in these challenging situations needs to be monitored closely by more experienced colleagues.

8 Service provision and management

Introduction

In the previous five chapters we have considered ethical issues clearly related to direct clinical practice, but there are wider issues that also warrant attention. This chapter therefore moves beyond a focus on interactions between clients and individual healthcare providers to a consideration of ethical issues at management level and the ethics of resource allocation. While the welfare of clients is at the heart of the issues portrayed in these scenarios, clients appear only as a remote and unidentified group with no input, under normal conditions, to decisions that will affect their lives.

Increasing healthcare costs have prompted a variety of approaches to rationalisation of services, most often at the level of within-system changes in how benefits are distributed. Such changes can often leave clinicians to work within untested systems and/or to implement unpalatable procedures.

The development of caseload management systems designed to increase throughput has in itself become a major focus for SLTs (see, e.g., the Maroondah Caseload Management System [Pertile & Page, 2003]). Speech and language therapy tasks in the assessment and intervention stages are increasingly delegated to volunteers, parents, school nurses or teachers. Delegation can be appropriate in terms of providing services in clients' natural contexts, training those who will most frequently interact with clients and widening the reach of speech and language therapy services. Delegation also, however, carries inherent risks. One common delegation is to have other professional groups screen on our behalf in nurseries and schools. The ethical implications of screening, a routine and seemingly innocuous practice, are highlighted in Scenario 8.1.

This is the only chapter in the book in which we consider private, as opposed to public, practice. In countries with parallel public and private health systems such as Australia and the USA, private practice represents a significant sector of the speech language therapy workforce: 43.1% in Australia (Lambier & Atherton, 2003) and 17% in the USA (American Speech-Language-Hearing Association

[ASHA], 2008c), although in both countries the majority of private practitioners work part-time in this sector. Private practice raises particular issues around governance and commercial integrity, as Scenario 8.2 illustrates. For the time being we return to the context of publicly funded health services in Scenario 8.1.

Scenario 8.1

Scenario 8.1 presents the minutes of discussions between a service director and a senior SLT about ways forward in managing an all too common situation where resource allocation constraints have prompted a prioritisation system to be put into place.

Northside Community Health Centre
Minutes of Meeting 22 May between Director of Allied Health (Haneef Ibrahim) and Senior SLT (Jennifer Smith) regarding New Caseload Management System for the SLT Department

Background to the meeting

Ms Smith explained to Mr Ibrahim that two factors had led to an unsustainable increase in waiting lists for SLT services. Not aware that budget cuts might arise in the near future, a year ago the area health service had run a very successful health promotion campaign encouraging parents to seek assessment for their children if they had any concerns about their child's school-readiness in the lead-up to the new school year. Apparently without prior consultation with senior staff, six months after the conclusion of the campaign, the health service Chief Executive Officer announced severe budget cuts. This resulted in shedding of 25% of allied health and community nursing staff across the service. This meant that the SLT department now had only three instead of four SLTs. Since then, the SLT department had experienced a dramatic increase in its waiting list. There were now more than 100 children waiting for assessment, and at least 60 who had been assessed and were awaiting therapy. The department had received a number of complaints from child care centres about SLTs no longer visiting the centres. Mainstream schools in the catchment area of the centre were unhappy that several children referred for special needs assessment funding reports prior to the end of the school year had not been assessed in time for funding to be secured for them for the new school year. Ms Smith explained that the SLT Dept was unable to continue to function with only three SLTs and that she had requested the meeting with the Director of Allied Health to present her case for an increased staffing level.

Mr Ibrahim explained that the budgetary crisis which had led to staffing cuts was not going to improve in the short term. In addition, responsibility for home monitoring of renal patients and palliative care patients had recently been moved from the local hospital to the health centre. This would require further small reductions in allied health staffing to fund increased community nursing levels. Mr Ibrahim felt that the only way forward in the short term was for the SLT Dept to change its caseload prioritisation strategies and models of service. He suggested that in the long term they would need to look at re-profiling the SLT service and consider the use of SLT assistants.

Ms Smith and Mr Ibrahim discussed core service obligations of the SLT Dept, the cost-effectiveness of current models of service and criteria for prioritisation of cases. New criteria and guidelines for policies for caseload management in the SLT Dept were agreed.

ACTION: SLT Dept to develop details of these prioritisation criteria and policies and forward to the Director for comment by the end of the quarter.

Types of service to be offered

It was agreed that the focus of clinic-based services will be on children not yet enrolled in formal schooling (i.e. children 0–5 years). Intervention for children with speech and language impairments will no longer be offered on an individual basis; all services for this caseload type must be offered in groups and parents must agree to be trained to participate in the group sessions. While the majority of services for preschool children will be clinic-based, SLTs will continue to provide a screening service to local preschools, kindergartens and day care centres on request, and will continue to provide workshops for teachers, carers and assistants on optimising speech and language development for children. Referrals will continue to be accepted as normal for clinic-based services for preschool children from parents, teachers and other health and social service professionals. Home-based services will no longer routinely be offered, and will occur only in the assessment stage for new referrals.

Because SLTs are not employed by the local schools, services will continue to be offered for school-aged children, but only at the clinic. These would mainly be assessments for special needs funding applications, children requiring follow-up intervention after surgery (e.g. cleft palate or other orofacial surgery, cochlear implants), and treatment for children whose condition would be likely to worsen without treatment (e.g. vocal abuse, stuttering). Mass screenings of all children starting school will no longer be offered. SLTs may go into local schools once per quarter on request from a school, to do a brief assessment of children identified by staff using a screening tool to be provided by the SLTs. Therapy will not be delivered on a one-to-one basis at schools. SLTs will provide class-based programming suggestions, and run workshops for teachers and teacher aides on working in classrooms with children with communication impairments. SLTs will continue to liaise and consult with Special Needs or Visiting Teachers for children receiving funding for disabilities.

Eligibility for clinic-based services

Prioritisation criteria for children attending the clinic will be developed around the following general principles:

▪ Preschool children take priority over school-aged children
▪ Children are eligible for clinic-based services if it can be shown that family and/or teachers will conduct home or school-based follow-up on therapy
▪ Therapy should be provided only for conditions for which an evidence base exists, demonstrating the potential for measureable improvements
▪ Children with frank medical conditions take priority over children with developmental conditions which may improve without intervention; in general terms this means that a hierarchy of priority might be:
  – Dysphagia and failure-to-thrive
  – Chronic conditions such as autism, hearing impairment, cerebral palsy, cleft palate

- Stuttering
- Vocal disorders
- Language impairments
- Speech impairments
- Developmental speech and/or language delay
▓ Children with more severe conditions take priority over children with mild impairments.

Amount of service to be offered in clinic-based services

For new referrals, assessment and report writing must be completed in a one-hour block. All children, regardless of condition or severity, will only be eligible for six weekly sessions of treatment in any one cycle of therapy. They may be offered a subsequent six-week cycle of therapy if improvement is demonstrated in the first cycle of therapy, and the condition remains severe.

Home and/or school programmes will be provided for children at the end of each therapy cycle.

Services to families who fail to attend two sessions in any block of therapy will be terminated and they will be placed back on the waiting list.

Next meeting

Mr Ibrahim and Ms Smith are to meet in two months time.

ACTION: Ms Smith to work with the SLT staff over the next two months to articulate prioritisation criteria and policies for the new caseload management system. Ms Smith to present a brief discussion paper on possible future use of SLT Assistants in the light of possible future reductions in full-time SLT positions.

Commentary on Scenario 8.1

Sharynne McLeod

Scenario 8.1 concludes with the action plan that the SLTs should prioritise their caseloads and limit speech and language therapy services to a maximum of 12 weeks of intervention (in the most severe cases), and prioritise *against* school-aged children, children with developmental (non-medical) conditions, children with speech and language delay, and so forth. There is no evidence base to support denial of health and education services to children with disabilities. Indeed I would suggest that the issues raised in this scenario need to be addressed at the level of international human rights, government, policy and professional associations rather than by a group of SLTs and their administrator.

Access to appropriate healthcare and education is a basic human right. There are many documents that incorporate the human rights of children, including the Convention on Rights of the Child (United Nations, 1989), the Salamanca Statement on the Right to Education (United Nations, 1994a), Standard Rules for the Equalization of Opportunities (United Nations, 1994b) and the Convention on the Rights of Persons with Disabilities (United Nations, 2006). These documents state that children have the right to extra assistance in order to participate fully in society. For example, Article 23.3 of the United Nations Convention on the Rights of the Child (1989) states:

> *Recognizing the special needs of a disabled child, assistance extended in accordance with paragraph 2 of the present article shall be provided free of charge, whenever possible, taking into account the financial resources of the parents or others caring for the child, and shall be designed to ensure that the disabled child has effective access to and receives education, training, health care services, rehabilitation services, preparation for employment and recreation opportunities in a manner conducive to the child's achieving the fullest possible social integration and individual development, including his or her cultural and spiritual development.*

Similarly, Article 25 of the United Nations Convention on the Rights of Persons with Disabilities (2006) states:

> *States Parties recognize that persons with disabilities have the right to the enjoyment of the highest attainable standard of health without discrimination on the basis of disability. States Parties . . . shall provide those health services needed by persons with disabilities specifically because of their disabilities, including early identification and intervention as appropriate, and services designed to minimize and prevent further disabilities, including among children and older persons.*

Communication disability in children is recognised by the World Health Organization (2007) and as such these international conventions should apply. Communication is an essential skill for functioning in today's society, where the majority of jobs require excellent communication skills. As Ruben (2000) suggests, a person in a wheelchair with excellent communication skills is far more employable than a fit, athletic person with poor communication skills. Ruben calculated that the unemployment rate for those unable to speak intelligibly (i.e. people with speech impairments and developmental speech delay who were listed as the lowest priority groupings in Scenario 8.1) is an astounding 75.6% and the cost of communication impairment is said to be between 2.5% and 3% of the US Gross National Product.

In comparison, the cost of achieving functional outcomes in communication ranges from US$2,000 to $11,325 per child, depending on the severity of the impairment (T. Campbell, 1999). Early intervention for children with communication impairment has been found to be effective in randomised controlled trials (RCTs) (Almost & Rosenbaum, 1998; M. Jones et al., 2005) and meta-analyses of interventions (Law, Garrett & Nye, 2003). However, if insufficient intervention is provided, then gains are not observed in community-based RCTs of intervention for expressive speech and language skills (Glogowska, Roulstone, Enderby & Peters, 2000).

'Speech and language development is intimately related to all aspects of educational and social development' (Law, Boyle, Harris, Harkness & Nye, 1998, p. 2). A systematic review of the literature indicates that children who do not receive intervention, or who begin intervention in the school years, can continue to have educational, occupational and social difficulties for at least 28 years (Law et al., 1998). Having a communication impairment can impact on educational outcomes in both the short and long term. Children with communication impairment generally require more school-based remedial assistance than their typically developing peers, and may achieve lower grades. They can have difficulty with mathematics and literacy, including difficulty with phonological awareness, spelling, reading comprehension and reading accuracy. Children with language impairment have been reported to be withdrawn in the playground and spend less time interacting with their peers when compared to typically developing children (Fujiki, Brinton, Isaacson & Summers, 2001) and are more likely to be bullied (Knox & Conti-Ramsden, 2003). Emotionally disturbed adolescents have a higher prevalence of communication impairment. Indeed Rosenthal (2007) reported that 'communication deficits constituted a central feature of emotional disturbance in adolescence' (p. 191). Incarcerated people, including young offenders (Bryan, 2004) and adult female prisoners (Olson Wagner, Gray & Potter, 1983), are also reported to have a higher prevalence of communication impairment.

Children with communication impairment are often *invisible* and *unheard*. Their disability is not physically obvious and their voices can be unintelligible. Advocacy for these children is limited. Parents are often unable to advocate effectively for their children as they may also have communication impairments, evidenced by the significant genetic transmission of such disorders. Teachers and SLTs are unable to advocate, as the policies within health and education departments frequently exclude children with communication impairment, particularly in countries such as Australia that do not have laws mandating access to services. Effective service provision and early intervention for children with communication impairment can lead to amelioration of communication impairment. It is therefore important that scenarios such as indicated in this chapter are not left at the local level for determination of short-term solutions. The ultimate cost to society of these decisions needs to be considered and SLTs should be supported by their professional associations, by governments and by policy makers to provide appropriate services through accountability to international human rights.

Sharynne McLeod, Professor, School of Teacher Education, Charles Sturt University, Australia

Commentary on Scenario 8.1

Sue Roulstone

Implementing budgetary reductions following health promotion campaigns

Implementing health service cuts in areas that have just been a focus of a health promotion campaign seems like crass incompetence or at least poor planning. The resultant increase in the SLT waiting list might perhaps have been predicted: the health promotion campaign has raised awareness of potential problems in children and expectations of support, where previously there were no concerns or expectations. The service is now unable to respond. Some might argue that at least families are now aware of a potential problem and can take alternative actions, and that it would be paternalistic only to raise awareness where there is a certainty of providing government services. So it seems that planning of the health service cuts by senior management has been poor; the full impact of the service cuts has not been considered with senior staff, who could no doubt have predicted the likely impact. Even if the cuts in this area were inevitable, some prior consultation might have allowed some alternative arrangements to be considered and communicated to families and other users.

A similar danger exists with the proposed screening programmes. Although there are plans to provide training for education and care staff and to see children in clinic, this will not necessarily address the individual concerns of a family whose child is identified by the screening process. Within the service, the provision of screening on request may seem like a way of delivering some level of service; however, it is far from clear that there has been a thorough analysis of the likely outcome and benefit for those undergoing the screening.

In the short term, the concern is to provide support for the families currently on the waiting list and in those contexts where lack of speech and language therapy response is further restricting provision for individuals (e.g. with reference to the special needs assessment). In the longer term, more coordinated strategic planning and a systematic analysis of the needs of families in that area are needed, using epidemiological literature as well as public consultation which can then guide service development.

Prioritisation of patient groups and conditions

These managers have decided to focus services on specified groups and to deny or restrict services to others. The challenge is whether there is an ethical way to take such decisions, since in prioritising one group over another we unavoidably value one life (or the quality of one life) above another. In this scenario, it seems that value judgements are being made that it is more important to care for patients with higher immediate risk (e.g. those needing dialysis) than those whose quality of life will be affected in the longer term (i.e. those with the communication disorders), to care for those at the end of their life rather than those just starting out. There also seems to be a belief that it is better to do good for a smaller number than to spread the service more thinly to reach a higher number. Cost-effectiveness is mentioned as a guiding principle, as is the evidence base and the ability to demonstrate the potential for measurable improvement.

The next difficulty then is: How do we measure benefit? How do we compare the benefit of intervention for a child with autism with that for a child who stutters? We are all aware of clients with relatively mild conditions, who seem disproportionately disabled by their condition or who can benefit hugely from a small amount of intervention. Any tools that we have for such purposes are still inexact.

In the current UK National Health Service, where services are free at the point of delivery, the need for rationing and prioritisation is probably inevitable. So prioritisation schemes and decisions about rationing emerge in an attempt to manage scarce resources. Having responded similarly myself back in the 1980s, I suspect such strategies are still viewed by professionals as ways to support professionals under pressure.

There is probably no right way to ration services – in the end the judgements we make are based on the values we attach to different outcomes and benefits.

Any attempt to ration services is likely to meet with opposition. My position, as a practitioner who values inclusive partnership approaches, would now be to involve all stakeholders in the decisions. There is also some evidence that partnership approaches improve the acceptability of decisions. So, a way forward would be through full engagement of stakeholders in order to arrive at consensus regarding the way to manage scarce resources. While we may worry that people will be demanding and unreasonable, research has shown that the public understand the need to ration healthcare, but object if it appears covert and inexplicit (E. Cross, Goodacres & O'Chathain, 2006). It is also important that stakeholders such as professional colleagues are fully engaged in the process so that the impact on their services, including cost implication, is fully appreciated.

Fairness and choice

This particular issue contains two challenges: firstly, the fairness of offering the same level of care irrespective of need; and, secondly, the ability of parents and children to influence the decision making that leads to their care, since all the services are pre-determined.

Offering the same initial service to all groups may seem like a way to ensure equality. However, it is difficult to argue that this principle will be served; in that case one would expect the same level of care for the same level of need, not irrespective of need. Furthermore, the service runs the risk of perpetuating or even precipitating further inequity for socially disadvantaged groups. For example, some would argue that for disadvantaged groups, more support is needed for the same healthcare problem (Braveman & Gruskin, 2003). Aspects of the new policy, such as termination of care after two failed attendances, are likely to increase inequity for families from disadvantaged backgrounds.

The single model of service also produces constraints in terms of parents' and children's ability to determine their own care, particularly since there appears to have been no consultation in the process of designing the care pathway. To constrain services in this way is to remove any freedom of choice for parents and children. For example, by offering services only in a clinic context, we fail to take account of parents' preferences and constraints.

When services are under pressure, providing clear parameters can support professionals' decision making and help them to feel back in control. However, the effect for families is likely to be the opposite – feelings of powerlessness (Roulstone, 2007).

As with the previous section, a way forward is to involve stakeholders in the design of a number of care pathways. In the absence of tools which can help us measure need in all its complexity, recognising patient preferences and stakeholder views can begin to build services that families and other stakeholder groups accept and support. And, although in this scenario some decisions have already been taken between managers, it is never too late to turn these over to stakeholder groups for discussion and evolution.

Sue Roulstone, Professor of Speech and Language Therapy, Faculty of Health and Life Sciences, University of the West of England, Bristol, UK

Scenario 8.2

Scenario 8.2, framed in the form of a memo from a Director of Allied Health Services to her Senior SLT, Khadija Rahman, also raises issues of resource allocation, but introduces concerns around fiscal management in private practice and the supervision of assistants.

From: t.nguyen@highlandshospital.net

To: k.rahman@highlandshospital.net

Date: 2 November 2008 18.55

Subject: Speech and language therapy service

Priority: urgent

Dear Khadija

I tried to phone you this afternoon but did not manage to make contact. Since the recent difficulty in recruiting a replacement to the speech and language therapy post, I am sure you have little time to spare for discussion of administrative issues. I therefore thought it best to set out in an e-mail some issues requiring urgent clarification. I have a meeting tomorrow at 3.00 p.m. with representatives of the major insurers underwriting rehabilitation input within the hospital and require a response to the queries below prior to that meeting. My secretary will be touch tomorrow morning to arrange a time for us to meet.

My concerns arise from a conversation earlier today with Rosa Delgado, whom I met by chance outside the canteen. As she has worked here for many years as a therapy assistant, I took the opportunity to ask how the department is managing with a reduced service. Her response suggested that the service had not in fact been reduced but had been expanded to cover the craniofacial patients from the recently opened craniofacial surgery unit. I must admit I find this situation difficult to reconcile with the current staffing levels.

My understanding is that while you continue to assess patients with aphasia, and to discuss with them the implications of your assessment, responsibility for ongoing therapy has been devolved to Rosa herself. According to Rosa she conducts the therapy with groups of patients using programmes and packages of resources available in the department, supplemented with materials that she has identified on the internet. No doubt her long experience of working with this client group has been of assistance to her in this regard.

I am aware of Rosa's reputation as a diligent and reliable SLT assistant. However, I have three primary concerns about this situation and I would appreciate clarification relating to each:

1. It does not seem feasible for SLT input to have expanded at a time of reduced staffing without significant modifications in type/level of service somewhere else in the service.
2. I would like to see the written records of supervision sessions between you and Rosa covering the period 1 September to the present. As I am sure you are aware, hospital policy requires 'regular, documented supervision of assistant duties and workload'.
3. Having not received notification to the contrary, I have continued to issue all invoices for speech and language therapy input for aphasia undertaken on an individual basis by a qualified speech and language therapist. The conversation described above would appear to be at odds with the content of these invoices.

I am sure I do not need to underline for you the potential seriousness of these issues, hence the decision to provide this information prior to discussion tomorrow.

Regards

Thuy Nguyen

Director of Allied Health

Commentary on Scenario 8.2

Sue Roulstone

In this scenario, the management and ethical issues are closely intertwined. Communication between management and staff, accountability for budgets, budget reporting and contract monitoring would be identified by a management consultant for further consideration here. Principles of good management and ethical management should coincide, but it is sometimes tricky to know where an issue crosses the line from bad management to unethical behaviour.

Management integrity

The integrity of our managers is the first issue. Focusing on the senior health service manager, the challenging question is: how far is this manager's behaviour an example of poor management and how far does it suggest a lack of integrity that makes it unethical? We might expect that a manager, behaving with integrity, would not jump to conclusions and formulate actions based on gossip obtained in the corridor. It was legitimate to have a conversation with the speech and language therapy assistant and to allow that the conversation has substance; it is *not* reasonable to react to the information obtained with a knee-jerk attack on the speech and language therapy manager without further clarification. The timing might also be considered unreasonable: an e-mail sent after-hours, requiring action first thing the next morning.

We can understand the anxiety of the senior manager – stumbling across unsettling information hours before an important meeting with insurers. It is to be hoped that this senior manager is looking to protect staff and patients, although it is also possible that self-protection is high on the agenda.

Before further action ensues, the facts need to be established in conversation with the speech and language therapy manager. It would be reasonable at this stage merely to inform the insurers that a situation of potential concern about service to patients had arisen and that the manager would be in touch with the insurers again within a defined time-scale. It is not clear from this scenario who holds budgetary responsibility, but clarity about that along with the speech and language therapy manager's responsibilities for communicating service changes to the senior manager would also be advisable to avoid similar surprises in the future.

Reductions in one service to develop another: robbing Peter to pay Paul

It appears that the level of qualified speech and language therapy input has been reduced for people with aphasia; this has occurred in the context of a new service for patients receiving craniofacial surgery and staff recruitment problems. Since it is not clear who holds responsibility for the budget in this scenario, it is therefore also not clear who would have responsibility for making such a decision. The senior manager clearly feels that this should not have happened. Should the speech and language therapy manager have refused to take on new demands and maintained existing provision? There are contractual arrangements here which should have governed the immediate decision and the process of changing provision, which I return to below. However, the underpinning decision about how best to respond to increasing demands in the context of limited resources is one that many managers face and has been discussed in Scenario 8.1.

Duty of care and levels of supervision

The conversation between the senior manager and the assistant has suggested that the levels of supervision received by the assistant are inadequate. The concerns here are about protection for the patient, and about how far the assistant is acting within the limits of her own competence, skills and knowledge. It is also about how far the supervising therapist is fulfilling her duty of care to patients on the caseload. That is to say, a speech and language therapy assistant is required to work under the supervision of a qualified therapist and that therapist retains the duty of care for those patients seen by the assistant. We may find it difficult to envisage harmful outcomes, but these may not be life-or-death situations. For example, they may take the form of inaccurate information for patients, inappropriate reassurance or providing activities that are of little benefit. Beyond the risk issues, this is clearly not helpful to the relationship between patient and the speech and language therapy department in terms of the quality of service being offered.

It is easy to see how such a situation might arise. Many managers are wary of developing an assistant role because of the difficulties of providing ongoing supervision for assistants in the context of staff turnover. Regular supervisory contact allows therapist and assistant to make explicit their respective roles and responsibilities and to make clear which routines are within the assistant's job description and which ones fall outside that responsibility. When the staffing changes and roles and responsibilities are shifted and where supervision is not maintained, there is a risk that the assistant is left with or takes on a higher level of responsibility than is allowed by her job description or level of training.

In terms of solutions, it is paramount that a suitable supervisory structure is in place. This includes the hospital policy which is in place to protect staff and patients from unsafe practice. The definition used here of 'regular, documented supervision' leaves room for considerable interpretation – once a year could arguably be termed as regular! Some longer-term solutions may also be appropriate. For example, the assistant in question is clearly valued by the team. Taking time to evaluate her skills and to re-evaluate her role in the department may lead to a more efficient use of her skills.

Commercial integrity

There is a final issue about how these services are being delivered. As ethical professionals, we have a responsibility to maintain commercial and financial integrity in our working lives. In this case, there is doubt that the contracted service is being delivered as specified. The senior manager is rightly anxious about this, particularly in the context of the visit next day from the insurers, who in this case are providing the funding for the service. The service agreement specifies that therapy should be provided by a qualified therapist, so to deliver the service via an unqualified assistant is fraudulent.

It seems that a breakdown in communication has occurred between the two managers. This could have occurred at a number of levels – in terms of understanding the contract specifications and limitations, who has budgetary control or who has responsibility for delivering services. Given that there is a speech and language therapy assistant who has been operating for a number of years in the department, one might also question the original contract – is the assistant's role recognised at all within the contract? No doubt it is possible to negotiate a contract which allows for more flexibility regarding the balance of qualified and unqualified care.

This scenario contains a number of inter-related issues that are tightly bound up with good management practice and good communication between the senior manager and the speech and language therapy manager. Many complaints received in the National Health Service are related to poor communication of one sort or another. It is ironic that we as SLTs suffer from that problem too.

Sue Roulstone, Professor of Speech and Language Therapy, Faculty of Health and Life Sciences, University of the West of England, Bristol, UK

Commentary on Scenario 8.2

Travis T. Threats

There are three perspectives from which to approach this scenario, involving legal, ethical, and moral issues. [Readers should note that the distinction between ethics – as professional regulation – and morality – as wider issues of right and wrong – used in this commentary contrasts with the absence of such a distinction elsewhere in the book. The issue of different terminology is discussed in Chapter 2.] Legal considerations are typically set at a lower bar than professional ethics. Legal guidelines set the minimum behavior – behavior that would be considered criminally negligent if not met. Legal rules do not enforce on professionals ethical standards, such as utilizing the latest in evidence-based practice. Ethical practices are thus not always reflected in laws, and it is possible for the law to be in conflict with ethics and morality.

Legal issues

Since legal issues are determined by cultures and governments, there is variability in the world over what constitutes an illegal act. For example, in some countries adultery can be illegal, while many countries would consider it immoral behavior but not subject to legal sanctions. The legal specification of the level and type of supervision of speech language assistants required varies by country, with the United

States specifying this relationship at the state level. For example, in some US states, speech language assistants are licensed by the state and thus have their own legal and ethical rules. However, in other US states, only speech language pathologists (SLPs) are licensed while the state recognizes speech assistants as working under the direction and supervision of SLPs. In this latter case, only the SLPs would have direct possible legal actions taken against them if the speech assistants they supervise are not competent or are of harm to clients. In other countries such as the UK and Australia, speech assistants are not licensed or their supervising SLPs put under such strict legal mandates. In these countries, the inadequate supervision of a speech assistant would be considered unethical but not illegal.

In the US, if the SLP does not demonstrate adequate supervision of the speech assistant, then the facility has violated both its legal and its professional ethical responsibility for its clients. Since legal requirements are concerned with minimum behavior, an SLP could meet a legal level of supervision but still not provide adequate supervision for a given speech assistant, especially if the speech assistant had limited clinical skills. The minimum documentation required by law might be occurring, but the spirit and ethics of the notion of supervision would be violated. The SLP could, for example, simply be signing the speech assistant's notes in the medical chart without really reading them or commenting on them.

The immediate legal issue in this scenario is the one raised by the Director of Allied Health: the issue being whether the speech assistant, or the department as a whole, is operating within the law. One possible legal problem is whether the speech assistant is operating within her scope of practice. A second legal problem is if the third-party payer assumes that the services are being provided under the direction of an SLP when patients are, in fact, being seen by a speech assistant without such direction. In this case, the third-party payer could argue that the billing was fraudulent and thus illegal.

Moral and ethical issues

Ethical rules provided by speech language pathology professional organizations around the world vary widely in their degree of specificity in terms of the relationship between SLPs and speech language assistants. In the US, for example, the ASHA Code of Ethics lists 14 specific things a speech assistant *may not* do, including developing or even modifying treatment plans, or providing any counseling with the client or family about the status of the therapy. In contrast, in countries such as Australia, the speech language pathology professional codes of ethics are about behaviors SLPs should aspire to, rather than listing specific prohibited behaviors in legalistic terms. These differences among countries are a reflection of overall differences in their healthcare cultures.

In this scenario concerning a speech assistant, there is a question as to what direction she is being given. She has stated that she uses material from the clinic as well as internet searches. Internet searches are not inherently good or inherently bad. For example, articles from many high-quality journals are available online. However, even if using journals, does this assistant have the ability to successfully interpret results to apply to her clients, a skill many licensed SLPs may not have? Importantly, can the assistant successfully discriminate between reputable sources and what are essentially dressed-up advertisements for specific products that discuss the 'research' supporting them? One troubling aspect is that the assistant does not list the SLPs themselves as a source of therapy ideas, because even a well-written diagnostic report cannot give enough information to appropriately plan and, more importantly, adapt therapy for effective intervention. Thus, according to a prescriptive code of ethics such as ASHA's, this assistant and her SLP may not be practicing ethically. In all countries, if the assistant is not being given proper direction, or even worse is making poor treatment decisions, then the SLPs and the facility are considered as behaving unethically.

Ethically it would be especially troublesome if the facility shifted these responsibilities to the assistant so that the SLP could see the possibly better reimbursed type of clients (or the clients viewed by the facility as more prestigious to serve). It has been argued that this shift has occurred in some US facilities, with more emphasis on dysphagia than on neurogenic language disorders.

The needs of the few versus the many: health economics ethics

In addition to this traditional view of ethics for provision of therapeutic services, there are the ethical and moral aspects to the determination of healthcare allocations. Ethics looks at a set of guidelines for a specific profession, while morality looks at larger issues of right versus wrong. Professional ethics and morality do not necessarily lead to the same solutions. For example, in the professional ethics of law, even the guilty have a right to a vigorous defense. However, what if the person is guilty of a violent crime? Morality says that he or she should go to jail, but a lawyer who purposely mishandled a case to make sure a client went to jail could lose his or her license on professional ethical grounds.

One of the latter steps in the evidence-based practice research continuum is to look at cost-effectiveness. From this viewpoint, if the same outcomes can be reached with less expense, then the less expensive option should be chosen because it would provide the greatest number of people services for the same given amount of financial resources. Looking at cost-effectiveness, unless one can show that the therapy provided by SLPs is better than that provided by assistants, then we cannot really say that it is unethical for assistants to provide treatment.

Experimental proof that SLPs produced better outcomes than the assistants (if available) would still leave open the ethical question of allocation of resources. The question could then be whether these better outcomes are worth the extra cost and possible restriction of services. Imagine a scale from 0 to 5 with 0 being no intervention-based improvement for persons with aphasia and 5 being the best possible outcomes from aphasia therapy. Using only SLPs, 100 persons with aphasia could reach an average level of 4, but 50 persons would not be able to receive services at all because of professional shortages. Using a combination of SLPs and assistants, all 150 people with aphasia could receive therapy with an average outcome score of 3. In the first scenario, only 100 people receive therapy, but there are better outcomes, presumably because SLPs provided all the intervention. In the second scenario, the 150 people who received therapy from SLPs and assistants had positive outcomes, albeit not as good as the first group. If we do the mathematics here, the first case with only SLPs treating achieves a sum of 400; with SLPs and assistants the sum is 450. In other words, the gain is greater for the population of people with aphasia in the second example.

A professional, and legal, assumption is made that SLPs provide better assessment and intervention than assistants as a result of the SLPs' education and directed practicum experiences as students. But others have argued that professional organizations are not always moral, because they work more to protect their own interests than to best represent their clients. A cynical view on this might lead to the comment that the only thing that people in the health fields (including us saintly SLPs) care about with respect to people with disabilities is getting paid to treat them. Speech language therapy professional associations often push for governments to mandate that services for persons with communication disorders be primarily limited to us or under our direction. If these associations do this because they fear that without legal protections unqualified persons would be providing inferior services, then they are demonstrating ethical and moral behavior. However, if these associations push for legal restrictions on provision of services to ensure their members' own employability, then they are both ethically and morally wrong. In fact, it could be argued that the most immoral acts are ones that wrap themselves in moral language for selfish purposes.

In summary, this case of whether the speech assistant is functioning ethically is open to varying legal, ethical, and moral considerations. If she is not competent and/or is poorly supervised, then professional ethical guidelines are being violated, regardless of whether a law has been broken. On the converse, she could be technically breaking the law as written in a given country, region, or state, but providing excellent clinical, and thus also ethical, service. Lastly, the professional associations could be accused of immoral behavior by restricting clients' access to speech assistants in order to protect their members' employability and salaries.

Travis T. Threats, Professor and Chair, Department of Communication Sciences and Disorders, Saint Louis University, USA

Discussion

Earlier chapters focused on ethical issues about and between individuals. This chapter discusses ethical issues in the management of resources and service delivery. We begin with a discussion of the ethics of screening.

Screening

In Scenario 8.1, the SLT manager proposes training others to screen children for speech and language impairment. In a paper entitled 'Is Screeningitis an Incurable Disease?' Shickle and Chadwick (2007) define screening as 'a selection procedure for further investigation, applied to a population of asymptomatic individuals, with no personal or family history to suggest that they are at a higher risk ... than the rest of the population' (p. 12). Wilson and Jungner (2007), in a much-cited report on medical screening for the World Health Organization, state that screening procedures 'sort out apparently well persons who probably have a disease from those who probably do not' (p. 11). The use of the word 'probably' highlights the need for 'subtle changes in ethical orientation' (Thompson et al., 2000, p. 165) required in thinking about screening. In fact, screening in general is rich territory for ethical debate and 'requires as much ethical justification as other . . . interventions' (Downie & Macnaughton, 2007, p. 97). Although screening programmes in speech and language therapy may not catch the headlines in the way that, say, genetic screening currently does, the implications of offering screening programmes, and the way they are delivered, are worthy of our consideration.

Screening instruments have variable sensitivity (the ratio of true positives to all those who have the condition) and specificity (the ratio of true negatives to all those who do not have the condition). In a systematic review of screening programmes for children with speech and language delay, screening instruments were found to have sensitivity between 17 and 100% and specificity between 45 and 100% (Nelson, Nygren, Walker & Panoscha, 2006). The age of children at screening also contributes to the ability of screeners to identify children with speech and/or language problems (de Koning et al., 2004; Mattson, Mårild & Pehrsson, 2001). Failure of a screening programme to identify children who have a problem is potentially harmful since they may miss out on receiving intervention. By contrast, wrongly identifying children as having problems may unnecessarily raise parental anxiety. That anxiety will be raised further if parents are then unable to access services for their children or if, having been alerted to a problem, they find the available intervention ineffective. Wilson and Jungner (2007) list 10 principles that a screening programme should meet and state that 'of all the criteria that a screening test should fulfil, the ability to treat the condition adequately, when discovered, is perhaps the most important' (p. 27). In contrast, if families of falsely identified individuals do manage to access services, this may waste valuable resources while SLTs determine that there is no problem after all. The usual ethical justification for screening is that it potentially benefits the majority of a specified population while risking harm to a smaller number of individuals. For healthcare professionals focused primarily on the care of individuals, this can be a difficult perspective to assimilate.

Informed consent is one of the central concepts of modern medical ethics. The generally accepted standard of information is that it should be adequate for the potential participant in a procedure to make a properly informed decision, but even this level of information is difficult to provide in relation to screening programmes. The involvement of large numbers of people makes it impossible to tailor information for any individual. It is also difficult to give an accurate picture of potential advantages and disadvantages, given the variations in specificity and sensitivity of screening instruments (as outlined above) and the unpredictability of any subsequent intervention. As a result, many screening programmes employ some level of implicit rather than explicit consent and/or a system of opting out rather than in. Whether these approaches constitute informed consent or paternalistic decision making on behalf of a population (as noted by Roulstone) is open to question.

A further ethical consideration in screening is that, as in Scenario 8.1, it can involve some level of delegation of SLT tasks, with associated obligations for training and supervising the people who take the tasks on. The ethics of delegation and supervision is discussed later in this chapter.

Although the speech and language therapy department in Scenario 8.1 can expect to save money if a screening programme previously administered by SLTs is transferred to education staff, service managers have an associated ethical obligation to anticipate the outcomes of screening and allocate resources appropriately, a subject to which we turn in the next section.

Resource allocation

The topic of resource allocation is both complex and controversial, and underlines the centrality of ethical issues to the field of healthcare. How can we distribute fairly the resources at our disposal? Are the resources at our disposal for healthcare a fair allocation of resources in total? Beauchamp and Childress (2007) provide an overview of four levels of healthcare resource allocation. Firstly, the comprehensive national budget of a country needs to be distributed among areas such as education, defence, roads, health, and so on. Then the health budget needs to be allocated between public health (e.g. infectious disease control programmes, accident prevention programmes) and individual healthcare. At the next level, many factors need to be weighed in determining which groups will receive healthcare; factors such as the prevalence of diseases and disabling conditions, costs of treatments, pain and suffering incurred by individuals with diseases or disabilities, impact on length and quality of life, and so on. This level of funding of categories of patients and types of services involves what are termed macroallocation decisions. Finally, microallocation decisions need to be made about resources (e.g. treatments, drugs) for individual patients. Both Scenarios 8.1 and 8.2 involve macro- and microallocation decisions.

A number of authors (e.g. Beauchamp & Childress, 2009; A. Campbell et al., 2001) have outlined six principles on which decisions about fair distribution could conceivably be based. These would allocate resources to each person according to (a) equal share, (b) need, (c) effort, (d) contribution to society, (e) merit and (f) free-market exchanges. Only the first two principles seem to be acceptable in the context of health.

People with ongoing healthcare needs, such as those with communication impairments, may not have the capacity to make sufficient effort and thus contribution to society to claim a share of healthcare services. They may also struggle to be accorded the merit (on the basis of their personal qualities) to claim a share. Further, where national health services exist, they are set up precisely to reduce the impact of free-market exchanges, in order to protect access to a 'decent minimum' (Beauchamp & Childress, 2009, p. 260) of healthcare. We are therefore left with 'equal share' and 'need'.

Allocating resources on the basis of everyone receiving an equal share ignores the fact that some people simply have more healthcare needs than do others.

It may also result in virtually nobody getting effective care, 'the jam being spread so thinly it can no longer be tasted' (Sim, 1997, p. 127). The alternative – to provide different levels of healthcare according to need – presents some challenges as well. Arbitrating between competing needs is inherently difficult at both macroallocation and microallocation levels. For example, placing restrictions on categories of people risks disadvantaging individuals within a category who could benefit from even small amounts of intervention. Such a result may be the outcome of the management decisions taken in Scenario 8.1. Some children with mild speech impairment might make significant progress quickly with a short period of therapy, reducing possible future impact on literacy, self-esteem, educational attainment and employment levels.

Access to healthcare, in the shape of speech and language therapy, could be seen as a 'right', which is the perspective taken by McLeod in her commentary on Scenario 8.1. She draws on the United Nations Convention of the Rights of the Child (1989) to claim that categorising children with (so-called) mild communication impairments as ineligible to receive services constitutes a denial of their human rights. This is also in line with the view expressed in the UK Bercow Review (Department for Children, Schools and Families, 2008) (discussed in Chapter 6) that 'communication is a fundamental human right' (p. 14). In relation to education and healthcare, rights tend to be contrasted with 'interests'. The United Nations Convention on the Rights of the Child (1989) posits education as a basic right, but only to the decent minimum of a basic primary school level. Beyond that level, the benefits that accrue to individuals from secondary education and above serve to place these levels of education within the domain of what are referred to as interests. Similarly, basic healthcare is generally seen as a right, Article 24b of the Convention specifically emphasising the provision of primary healthcare. Beyond that basic level, it becomes an interest (Berglund, 2007). National (universal) health systems attempt to meet the rights of citizens to a basic level of health care, also providing some services significantly beyond this level. Private health systems cater to the 'interests' of those who can afford care beyond the basic level. The challenge for professions and health service managers is in deciding between rights and interests.

An alternative ethical view of the right to resources also involves a balance, this time between what is 'unfair' and what is 'unfortunate'. Philosophers such as Rawls (2007) and Daniels (2007) discuss whether society has an obligation to attend to conditions which are unfairly disadvantaging, but not necessarily to those which could be considered merely unfortunate. As with the contrast between 'rights' and 'interests', the perception of 'unfair' and 'unfortunate' may differ between the speech and language therapy profession and society as a whole. SLTs are likely to see the children with speech impairments in Scenario 8.1 and the people with aphasia in Scenario 8.2 as unfairly disadvantaged rather than unfortunate.

A major approach to resource allocation attempts to balance costs, benefits and effectiveness of intervention by means of cost-benefit analyses (comparing the cost of an intervention with the expected outcomes/benefits) and cost-effectiveness analyses (comparing alternatives to achieving a specified outcome). The most commonly used cost-effectiveness analysis measure is the quality-adjusted life year (QALY). In this system, numerical weighting is given to years of healthy (or unhealthy) life and to the quality of life experienced in those years. Hence, QALYs 'bring length of life and quality of life into a singe framework of evaluation' (Beauchamp & Childress, 2009, p. 231). Underlying this approach is the notion of providing the best health outcomes for the most people overall.

If QALYs were to be applied to Scenario 8.1, a different management decision would probably be made. Resources would not be withdrawn from children with speech impairment, since their age, general health and the effectiveness of early speech and language therapy would predict a large number of quality years ahead of them. In Scenario 8.2, on the other hand, QALYs could be used to support the decision to move resources from people with aphasia to those requiring craniofacial surgery, as both age and chronic disability would count against older people with aphasia. One of the major ethical criticisms of QALYs is that they inherently discriminate against older people. One attempt to address this limitation is a modification called the Disability Adjusted Life Year (DALY), in which a system of discounting lessens the effect of age (Arnesen & Nord, 1999).

The various ethical viewpoints and resource allocation approaches discussed above still beg the question of who decides what constitute rights, interests, (un)fairness, (mis)fortune and quality of life. One approach to making decisions about such allocations involves engaging people in prioritising services that are important for them in their communities (Beauchamp & Childress, 2009). This may involve asking communities to rank services by social value. Roulstone suggests we use epidemiological information to help communities make informed decisions about what they want. For example, establishing a community speech and language service in a community with a high number of young female sole parents with preschool-age children would suggest that early intervention services, preschool or nursery programmes and services in schools might take priority over services for adults with communication impairments, especially if another nearby service can provide them. In contrast, in a community with a high number of retirees, the health service might prioritise stroke rehabilitation services, community-based stroke groups and programmes for people with progressive neurological diseases. Roulstone suggests that people are more likely to accept allocation decisions if they experience a sense of ownership and control over those decisions.

This grassroots approach, while consultative and potentially sensitive to the perceptions of consumers, raises ethical concerns about who is determining what on behalf of others. In this sort of approach the voices of people with illness and disabilities, infants, the elderly and the disadvantaged may struggle to make themselves heard over those of other more powerful and vocal sectors of the community. Indeed, can non-disabled people make legitimate judgements about the value of services for people with disabilities? As Sim (2007) notes, 'the fact that a life may not seem to be worth living to society at large does not necessarily mean that it is not worth living for the person whose life it is'(p. 125). This sentiment can be extrapolated to quality of life and its measurement across the board.

The fact that judgements are routinely made about care for people with disabilities by those without places an obligation on SLTs to advocate for people with communication impairments. Such advocacy is clearly recognised as part of our role and is stated in some codes of ethics (e.g. Speech Pathology Australia, 2000), despite the lack of an evidence base for this role. SLTs should also lobby for the inclusion of people with disabilities in organisations or groups that make decisions about people with disabilities, such as local health service boards. What is striking in both Scenarios 8.1 and 8.2 is that resources are being moved from those with little (political) voice – children with speech impairments and people with aphasia – to those with potential voice, political clout and heavyweight professional backing (adults with renal and palliative care needs in Scenario 8.1 and requiring craniofacial surgery in Scenario 8.2).

Delegation and supervision

Both Scenarios 8.1 and 8.2 involve delegation of some sort, and Scenario 8.2 features an apparent failure of supervision. In Scenario 8.1, the Senior SLT intends to delegate initial screening for speech and language difficulties to teachers in schools. The teachers will use a screening procedure provided by the SLTs. Issues associated with screening have been discussed earlier in this chapter. In Scenario 8.2, speech and language therapy services to people with aphasia have been delegated by the SLT to the speech and language therapy assistant (SLTA).

Delegation of tasks to assistants and other professionals is a routine part of speech and language therapy practice but is not without risks. This is reflected in the various position statements and guidelines on training, deployment and supervision of assistants (see, e.g., the ASHA guidelines 2004 and various codes of ethics [e.g. Speech Pathology Australia, 2000]). Some professional associations such as ASHA severely restrict the scope of delegation, whereas other countries allow delegation to a range of volunteers and other professionals such as teachers.

To date there has been relatively little discussion in speech and language therapy of the nature of any risks and whether they outweigh the benefits. The risks of delegation are of course more foregrounded in the medical literature (see, e.g., Cook, 1980; Stranjalis, 1996), where errors may be associated with injury, death and litigation when delegated tasks are not carried out sufficiently well. Discussion of issues and risks in delegation has recently started to appear in other allied health literature. Mackey (2007) reflects on the delegation in occupational therapy with the introduction of assistants in the UK National Health Service. Qualitative data analysis of focus group interviews with assistants, supervisors, managers and clients identified lack of clarity about how tasks were delegated and ambiguity about who took responsibility for the outcomes of services provided. There were also tensions around recognition of qualifications and competence between levels of staff. A clear implication of this study is that clarity about team roles and delegation processes needs to be established in order to ensure that service users receive the most appropriate care from the most appropriate practitioner. Findings such as these compel SLTs to consider what, how and why we delegate and to whom.

It is obvious that the major risk in delegation of speech and language therapy tasks lies in delivery of less than optimal services to clients. At worst, real harm may ensue to clients who receive inappropriate treatment, or who are not identified (e.g. by screening) and fail to access services before their communication impairment impedes subsequent development.

Supervision of those to whom we delegate is essential to protect professional integrity, client care and the person to whom we delegate. In Scenario 8.2 Khadija appears to have failed to provide supervision of her SLTA, Rosa, because of workload issues. The ASHA guidelines on delegation demarcate clearly that assistants should not carry their own caseload, this being the responsibility of SLTs. Khadija would almost certainly be deemed in violation of various codes of ethics. While action may well be taken against Khadija by her employer and by her professional association if she is found to have been negligent in the provision of supervision, it is worth attempting to understand why this failure of supervision occurred. Increasing caseloads and attrition in the health workforce worldwide mean Khadija would not be the first SLT to fail to provide regular and appropriate supervision to workplace assistants.

Although the expectation is that the SLT's time in direct service delivery will decrease in proportion to the time required for supervision of assistants or staff, such time can be very hard to secure. Clinicians focused on client care may prioritise clients over other duties such as administration or supervision. Further, many SLTAs and indeed volunteers such as those trained to provide supported conversation for people with aphasia (Kagan, Black, Duchan, Simmons-Mackie & Square, 2001) are clearly competent. If time is short, and the delegation appears to be progressing well, SLTs may not remember that supervision in the workplace has as ensuring role as well as an enabling role (Morton-Cooper & Palmer, 2000). Assistants and volunteers and indeed staff performing competently and developing their knowledge and skills independently may not require 'enabling' to do so. However, they may still legally and ethically require 'ensuring' that the delegated tasks are being done to the required standard with the required documentation.

An additional factor to consider in failure of supervision is the role of interpersonal dynamics in the workplace. Assistants and junior staff may be older and even more experienced with the caseload than the fully qualified professional. This is possibly the situation Khadija finds herself in with her assistant Rosa. It can be challenging to override age and experience barriers to enact the authority vested in workplace supervisors. Moreover, teams can develop a web of personal and professional relationships that can further complicate supervisory relationships (Kadushin, 1968).

A final factor to consider in failure of supervision is the knowledge and skill of the supervisor pertinent to the supervisory process. Supervisors are often unprepared for their role and unable to access workplace support or professional education for the execution and development of their skills in supervision (Ferguson, 2005). All these factors will need to be considered by Khadija's manager when they meet to explore the facts of the situation and decide how to act, to deal with both the current situation and to ensure such situations do not arise again in her department.

Protection of interests

Protection of interests may not seem, at first sight, a concept closely associated with the provision of healthcare. 'Joint working is essential' (Department for Children, Schools and Families, 2008, p. 6) is a mantra of many modern health services, and multi-, inter- and even transdisciplinary team formats are seen as the embodiment of this ideal. Scenarios 8.1 and 8.2 give us cause to ponder the subtleties of professional boundary protection and to examine whose interests are being served. In the discussion of private therapy in Chapter 5 we saw how professionals are theoretically expected to put the patient's interests above their own. However, health work is never this straightforward.

In Scenario 8.1, Ms Smith, the speech and language therapy manager, is under pressure to reorganise service priorities and effectively exclude some children from services. Although Ms Smith may well be driven by a desire to provide speech and language therapy services for all, she will also want to avoid conflict with her manager, not least because conflict is time-consuming and energy-draining. Despite the fact that the interests of some client groups will not be served if she acquiesces, she also has to factor in the need to protect her service from even further cuts and the need to maintain a working relationship with the other professionals around her. Ms Smith will need moral and professional courage to withstand the pressure to reduce services, particularly given that the other pressures may constitute a line of least resistance.

Similarly, both the SLT and the Director of Allied Health are struggling to protect a variety of interests in Scenario 8.2. The director may immediately have recognised the implications for the hospital's contract with the insurer if services have not been delivered as contracted and if faulty billing practices have ensued. At least part of her response will come from the knowledge that she herself might become the focus of ethical, and quite possibly legal, attention. In countries such as the UK and Canada, where the predominant model of healthcare is a national health service funded by tax payers but free at point of delivery, managers do not typically have to grapple with the complexities of private health insurance, compensable clients and reimbursement for services provided. However, such services prevail in the US, and Australia has a mix of a publicly funded national health service and private health care. Ethical complaints relating to fraudulent or inaccurate billing are frequently brought before ASHA's Ethics Board (ASHA Ethics Board Chair, personal communication, November 2003).

Scenario 8.2 raises a third aspect of protection of interests in relation to the deployment of SLTAs. We have already discussed some of the challenges of supervision, but Threats asks us also to consider the possibility that professional protectionism might underlie surface arguments about public safety.

Threats suggests it may be immoral for professional associations to mandate against delegation of tasks to lesser trained staff in the absence of evidence that fully qualified professionals can do a better job of service delivery. He makes the argument that if providing access to services for all potential clients lies at the heart of what motivates us as professionals, then we may need to look at the costs and benefits. In other words, what are the potential risks of less qualified personnel delivering services to a larger sector of the population?

A growing body of research into the effectives of volunteers and assistants suggests that, with appropriate training by SLTs, both groups may be able to provide effective services for people with communication impairments. For example, Kagan et al. (2001) found that trained volunteers were able effectively to support conversation skills of people with aphasia. More recently, Boyle, McCartney, Forbes and O'Hare (2007) compared what were described as current models and levels of SLT service with the following modes of service delivery: SLT providing direct individual therapy; indirect individual therapy delivered by SLTA; direct group therapy from SLT; and indirect group therapy from SLTA. Results of primary outcome measures revealed no significant post-intervention differences between direct and indirect modes of therapy, or between individual and group modes of service delivery. However, intervention studies of this kind have complex design and analysis features, and secondary outcome measures did reveal better gains in expressive language from direct therapy. As always, replication is required before we can be confident in the results of one study, but the results of these and similar studies should caution SLTs about untested assumptions driving resource allocation and service delivery decisions.

Threats in fact asks us to consider not only whether SLTAs or other support personnel can be as effective in some circumstances as qualified clinicians. He also questions whether, even if the evidence were to suggest that service delivery by SLTAs is less effective than that provided by SLTs, the provision of such a service to a greater number of people actually renders it the more ethical use of resources. In circumstances of high economic pressure and development of consultancy models in general, the SLT profession will need to work hard to balance these resources to provide the best services to the largest number of people.

Summary

This chapter has moved the focus away from direct services and interactions between clients and healthcare providers to a consideration of the ethics of management in speech and language therapy services. Rationing of healthcare resources and prioritisation of client groups and individual clients seem inevitable consequences of contemporary healthcare. This chapter encourages SLTs to consider the ethics of decisions made by their managers and indeed by themselves as they prioritise and arrange their workloads. There is a vast literature, some of which we have summarised, on specific procedures (such as QALYs) and political approaches (such as stakeholder consultation) relevant to the challenges of resource allocation.

One way of managing decreasing resources for speech and language therapy has been by increasing the use of screening, as described in Scenario 8.1. This raises ethical considerations in terms of whether people have any choice in participating, whether the instrument can actually identify the right people for intervention and whether there actually *is* any intervention available.

Delegation, a further response to resource restrictions, carries with it obligations for close attention to the maintenance of service standards. As we saw in Scenario 8.2, it can also raise the interesting – though potentially uncomfortable – topic of protection of professional interests as SLTs consider the more widespread use of assistants and volunteers.

9 Common themes and emerging trends

Introduction

We begin this final chapter by reflecting on the issues that are shared across client groups and service settings. Although we have used specific clinical scenarios to prompt discussion, many of the themes are also found in other circumstances, though they may manifest differently. This reflection is followed by a discussion of emerging trends, both within speech and language therapy and in the wider healthcare environment. We round off both the chapter and the book with some thoughts on the teaching and learning of ethics.

Common themes

In the following we consider a select few examples of issues common to various scenarios in the preceding chapters.

Talking things through

In the opening chapters of the book we referred to the need to get more discussion of ethical issues out in the open. There are many situations in the scenarios either where clinicians are seen talking through their thoughts and feelings with colleagues or where it looks as though they would benefit from doing so.

  Sophie, the student in Scenario 7.1 (p. 126), is concerned about the actions of the volunteer with whom she is on placement and about the implications of any action she takes for her own assessment report. Chinwe, in Scenario 7.2 (p. 133), a newly qualified therapist trying to get to grips with the unfamiliar challenge presented by someone with Parkinson's disease, checks out some of her doubts in e-mail correspondence with her friend from college. Jennifer Smith, the speech and language therapy manager in Scenario 8.1 (p. 148) faced with significant service restrictions, could do with talking through her options as she seeks some form of plan.

For students and those starting out in the profession, the benefit of discussing ethical issues can sometimes take the form of relief, knowing that other, more experienced clinicians have made errors and are willing to air them in public. For managers and students alike, talking things through can provide a way of breaking out of the vicious circle of one's thoughts and values.

In Chapter 4 we suggested that clinicians working in multidisciplinary teams might not automatically know in detail what responsibilities each team member thinks each of the other team members has, and that this inevitably leads to gaps and overlaps in service. Similarly, it is difficult to understand the values held by other clinicians without asking them. For instance, how many of us could predict with any accuracy exactly how a selection of our colleagues would respond to the opening question in Scenario 4.1 (p. 57): 'What would you do if Poppy was your daughter?' More importantly, how can we be sure that what we predict is actually how colleagues would answer? Yet, if the service that we provide is going to be consistent, the response that Anthea receives to this question should not really depend on who she asks. Only by discussing these issues when – and preferably before – they arise can people understand and manage their colleagues' views. As we discussed in Chapter 2, the broad statements made public in codes of ethics tell us about professional values in only the most general terms and cannot prevent different clinicians giving conflicting responses to the same questions.

Although the various people in the scenarios could benefit from talking through ethical issues, there is no getting away from the fact that discussion can be time-consuming. If it wasn't, it is likely that the issues themselves could be resolved rapidly anyway. Nevertheless, as illustrated by Vesna (Scenario 6.2, p. 108) pondering a work issue while sitting at her kitchen table, dealing with situations that are ethically uncomfortable inevitably takes time in one way or another.

Maintaining confidentiality during the process of checking things out is sometimes more difficult than it appears on the surface. Chinwe needs to be very careful in discussing clinical issues within e-mails. The widespread use of legal cautions within e-mails is no guarantee that they will not be misdirected or intercepted. Many organisations prohibit or restrict the inclusion of specific client information in electronic communications systems, and some ethicists are suggesting that it is time to investigate the use of passwords, perhaps in the way they are used in commercial transactions, for telephone consultations in the first instance and, by extension, presumably for other telehealth applications in due course (see discussion below) (Sokol & Car, 2006). Even carefully anonymised discussion can be deciphered by other people. For example, writing on the subject of ethical challenges in the field of mental health and hearing impairment, Gutman (2005) points out that '[t]he Deaf community is closely knit, so clinicians may find that maintaining confidentiality and avoiding multiple relationships requires great delicacy and tact' (p. 174).

Of course, discussion is no guarantee of either ethically robust action or peace of mind. Many discussions and decisions end up not pleasing everybody. The discussion in Chapter 6 about making decisions on behalf of children highlights the importance of taking into consideration the child's place in the family and, indeed, in the wider social environment. Decisions that ostensibly benefit one child but disadvantage siblings stand a chance of backfiring by indirectly disadvantaging the child in question as well. Some ethical challenges push people's values too far, such as those outlined in the discussion of the role of conscience in Chapter 3, and thus cannot be resolved to everyone's satisfaction. As Marshall writes in her second commentary for Chapter 6:

> [I]t is important for SLTs to distinguish between situations for which they need increased knowledge and experience and situations which they handled well but which leave them feeling uncomfortable because there is no resolution that would satisfy all parties.

This may be an appropriate point to revisit the issue of conscience briefly, since it tends to come to the fore in situations where people cannot find a consensus view. The discussion earlier in the book (Chapter 3) was based on refusal of non-oral feeding and the possibility of SLTs feeling obliged to discontinue their involvement on the basis of their conscience. Since the discussion was couched in terms of 'conscientious objection', it may seem that it would be a rare occurrence in speech and language therapy, and at this relatively dramatic level that is probably true. However, the concept is relevant at other levels. For example, a recent discussion in the medical ethics literature has tackled the potentially contentious issue of ideological (e.g. religious) symbols in the workplace. The personal beliefs of many health workers encourage or in some cases require them to wear or display items that are representative of religious faith. And yet, according to Schuklenk (2006):

> The issue at hand is how the patient perceives and interprets the symbols…and the negative consequences of withholding vital lifestyle or health-related information for fear of disapprobation from the doctor or other health professional. (p. 1)

Schuklenk further suggests that health professionals should leave all ideological symbols outside the workplace. This is clearly an issue about which comprehensive agreement would be difficult to achieve, but it needs talking about nonetheless. It is also relevant to the emerging issues discussed later in this chapter in the sense that it is part of recent discussion in medical ethics circles and is entirely relevant to speech and language therapy as well, which suggests that the profession should be looking outwards to get an idea of ethical issues emerging close by.

Roles and boundaries

Several of the scenarios involve people pondering whether a course of action is within the boundaries they consider appropriate for their role, or other people challenging those boundaries. Vesna (Scenario 6.2) is contemplating whether to take up the case of Sam and his mother despite the fact that Sam is no longer on her caseload. This possibility has been brought to her attention by Sam's mother outside work hours and outside the work location. Andrew (Scenario 4.2, p. 63) has multiple responsibilities to his client Kieran, but the care workers are challenging the legitimacy of Andrew concerning himself with the topic of Kieran's sex life.

Should the SLT trying to engage Della and her mother in the therapy process (Scenario 6.1, p. 99) expand her role to health promotion in general? In Chapter 5 we alluded to the Whatever It Takes model (Willer & Corrigan, 1994) for community brain injury rehabilitation, which is an attempt to reduce the effect of fixed professional roles on delivery of what the client actually needs. Doing whatever it takes may potentially be a better way of providing a client-centred service, but it can present clinicians with serious challenges to their professional boundaries.

The difficulties of professional boundary definition are mirrored by a lack of clear definition of client boundaries. Dean's priorities after his brain injury (Scenario 5.2, p. 84) are at odds with some of his mother's priorities for him. It is not clear that Julianna's needs (Scenario 5.1, p. 78) are being well represented by her husband. Meanwhile, in Scenario 7.1, Elsie's needs as her dementia becomes more severe may not match those of her husband Harold, himself struggling with disability. In these cases individual client autonomy is not easy to accommodate within a broader philosophy of integrated family services. As ever, these issues can only be dealt with by clinicians being aware of the potential for them to arise and negotiating with all relevant stakeholders.

Power and control

Though it may not always feel like it in clinical practice, SLTs routinely find themselves in positions of psychological and practical power, often in direct proportion to the reduction in power and control experienced by clients. Andrew (Scenario 4.2) is the primary selector of signs for his client Kieran and is in a position thereby to exert control over the content of Kieran's communication. From a different perspective, Nadia, supervisor of Sophie's clinical placement (Scenario 7.1), has significant power in relation to allocating assessment marks and writing up a placement report. The man lying in bed in Scenario 3.2 (p. 43) appears to have very restricted control over decisions about his nutrition as he listens to his daughter and the SLT discussing the issue.

Of course, even senior SLTs do not sit at the top of some organisational tree dispensing or withholding power and control. They themselves are subject to controlling influences by other people. Khadija Rahman's deployment of the SLT assistant in Scenario 8.2 (p. 155) has placed her in a vulnerable position in relation to the Director of Allied Health. Jackie Delaney in Scenario 3.1 (p. 36) has responsibility for the actions of her staff and will have to answer to the hospital medical establishment in the form of Dr Giuliani. This recognition of the salience of power and control in healthcare takes us back to the discussion in Chapter 2 which acknowledged Brody's (2002) argument that the concept of power is an essential component in any system of ethics.

Language as speech act

Throughout the book we have tried to emphasise the critical role of language in healthcare ethics in general and speech and language therapy ethics in particular.

We started with an example in Chapter 1 of the ethical ramifications of the single word 'yet'. Several of the commentators in the book have written about the influence of word and phrase selection in the scenarios presented in report format. The SLT's reflective log on the interaction with Della's mother (Scenario 6.1) contains some subtly negative connotations. The hospital report about Dean after his brain injury (Scenario 5.2) is in similar vein. Togher et al. (1997) demonstrate how changes occur in the way people, including family members, talk to someone after brain injury, underlining the need for SLTs to be vigilant to the nuances of their language.

Another facet of the importance of exact choices of words has been seen in the responses that professionals make to questions or how they phrase explanations. We have discussed the factors Susan (Scenario 4.1) has to take into consideration in her response to a direct question about what she would do in similar circumstances. A parallel example of the subtleties involved in responding to direct questions, involving the same Mrs Davies as in Chapter 1, comes at the very end of this chapter.

Many of the common issues we have identified in this section will no doubt continue to be important as the profession deals with the emerging ethical issues discussed in the next section.

Emerging ethical issues in speech and language therapy practice

In this section we focus on issues that appear to be at the forefront of the profession's thinking at the moment and consider implications for future practice. This discussion is based in part on a workshop conducted by one of the authors (LM) at the 2007 Speech Pathology Australia National Conference held in Sydney. About 60 SLTs working in small groups were asked to discuss what they saw as emerging ethical issues for the profession. A summary of these issues is provided in Box 9.1. The majority of contributions focused not on individual client/healthcare provider interactions but on larger systemic issues. Some of these issues are used to frame a discussion of demographic, social, technological and systemic trends and their relationship to ethics.

Emerging ethical issues for Australian Speech Pathologists

1) Tension between service policies and values of profession
   Medical focus on saving lives versus quality of life
   Organisational health and safety risk management versus client quality of life
2) Resource allocation and prioritisation
   Restricting rights of others by focusing on particular service areas
   Narrowing of services for some groups (e.g. fluency, voice)

Families forced to seek private therapy due to decreased service in public sector
Prioritisation: clinician choice versus service direction
Early intervention: behaviour problems priority over speech and language
Decision making uneven across sectors e.g. acute/disability
One-size-fits-all decisions within sectors
Tightening of eligibility for services related to age
Difficulty engaging with clients affected by limitations of service
Push for discharge versus completion of episode of care
Services to clients of non-English-speaking backgrounds
3) Workforce issues
    Access to continuing professional development.
    Supervision standards for rural and remote SLTs
    Use of allied health assistants and support workers:
        e.g. role clarification, training, standards for practice, accountability
    Private practice standards
    Discipline specific versus multidisciplinary student placements
4) Service user and service delivery
    Consultancy role for SLTs
    Expansion of roles in workplace in areas of e.g. care planning, advocacy
    Evidence-based practice:
        Time limits imposed not based on evidence
        Reliability of evidence
        Assimilating multiple sources of evidence
        Lack of evidence generally
        Ethical responsibility to research areas with restricted evidence

Healthcare values

SLTs in the workshop described increasing underlying tension between the values underpinning new service policies in their workplaces (such as those outlining prioritisation of client groups) and what they believed to be the values of the speech and language therapy profession. Although the workshop did not explore exactly what these professional values were perceived to be, the SLTs were very critical of management policies which they saw as overriding client-focused care. Codes of ethics for SLTs highlight their duties to employers and colleagues as well as to clients. The fulfilment of duties to different parties can make for uncomfortable ethical territory. For example, SLTs in many countries are bound by legislation not to publicly criticise their employers or to disclose information that might reflect poorly on their employer or the services provided. Public discussion of unsatisfactory management policies may be one way of meeting duties to clients, yet doing so may contravene the duty to employers and have legal ramifications for the staff involved.

The discrepancy between organisational and professional values is exemplified by an increasing organisational focus on risk management, which was seen to sometimes reduce clients' autonomy and quality of life. The example given by one workshop participant was of a group home for adults where a client had successfully requested scotch whisky thickened to an appropriate level for his dysphagia. The decision was subsequently revoked as a health and safety risk to the organisation. Increasing client complexity, together with increasing litigation and indemnity costs, will quite possibly see risk management policies further curbing aspects of speech and language therapy practice and client autonomy. The tension around this issue arises in part because the relationship between SLTs and clients is sometimes founded on the support provided by clinicians specifically to encourage clients to take *more* risk. The social communication tasks undertaken during therapy by people with dysfluency, for example, are inherently psychologically risky.

Resource allocation

The largest number of concerns expressed in the workshop related to resource allocation and prioritisation of clients. As with the other issues, these may not be solely new concerns, but the detail involved changes accompanying developments in healthcare. Some of the concerns related to economic drivers of resource allocation in healthcare, the contexts and challenges of which were discussed in Chapter 8. Though not raised in the workshop or the scenarios in Chapter 8, these concerns are also of increasing importance in countries with healthcare systems predominantly funded privately via insurance. For the system in the USA, for example, the ethical and political dilemmas posed by people without health insurance are very pressing indeed.

The SLTs in the workshop gave examples of different client groups missing out on service or having access to limited services only (see Box 9.1), clearly illustrating what they saw as ethical dilemmas in prioritisation. Further, they were critical of decisions made about the amount or timing of service that were based not on evidence but on cost (as illustrated in Scenario 5.1). One particular example concerned the use of age as a criterion in determining eligibility for service. As discussed in the introduction to Chapter 7, the world's population as a whole is ageing. In all but the 50 least developed countries, rapid population ageing is expected (United Nations, 2007), with a consequent increase in demand for speech and language therapy services, where they exist. Increased longevity is associated with increased prevalence of progressive neurological diseases such as Parkinson's disease, making a range of demands on SLTs who may be trying to provide services to such people as part of a generalist caseload (as in Scenario 7.2).

Another factor likely to have an impact on speech and language therapy resources is the ongoing increase in survival rates of people with disabilities and complex medical needs. For example, very low birthweight neonates now routinely survive neonatal intensive care, but at a potential cost in terms of immediate disability or, for example, language and learning disability later in development (Hack, 2007; Moster, Lie & Markestad, 2008). Advances in neurosurgery after traumatic brain injury and the use of pharmaceuticals which prolong life are further examples of this trend. The SLTs in the workshop reported concerns about the quality of life that ensues for people living with severe and complex disabilities; these concerns are likely to be shared by health professionals around the world who are responsible for habilitation and rehabilitation of clients of all ages.

A relatively unknown quantity in terms of predicting future influences on resource allocation comes from the field of genetics. The last decade has seen announcements of discoveries of genes linked to communication disorders. For example, mutation of the FOXP2 gene has been linked to difficulty in speech and language development (Marcus & Fisher, 2003), though the full picture is likely to be complex (Meaburn, Dale, Craig & Plomin, 2002), and IRF6 gene disruption has been linked to nonsyndromic cleft lip and palate (Scapoli et al., 2003). Advances in genetics have implications for clinical practice in speech and language therapy. For example, how might these developments influence our diagnosis, assessment and referral of people with communication disabilities? How might these and future developments influence the advice and support we give to parents for whom the SLT might be the first point of contact with the health sector?

The healthcare workforce

Not only do we have an ageing population requiring and expecting a high level of healthcare, but many countries also have an ageing healthcare workforce. For example, an Australian Government report makes the following assessment of the situation:

> Service providers will be seeking to replace greater numbers of retiring workers, and to secure additional labour to meet accelerating demand, in an environment where growth in effective labour supply is expected to be slower than population growth. (Productivity Commission, 2005, p. xviii)

One response to such workforce shortages in developed countries has been to recruit aggressively from developing countries, a practice which strips health professionals from countries already critically short of health staff and raises significant ethical issues of international responsibility.

Another potential response to workforce shortages is to increase the use of support workers. Scenario 8.2 portrayed some of the benefits and risks of delivering services via assistants. Increases in the deployment of assistants and generic health workers could potentially present the profession with an opportunity to extend the reach of speech and language therapy services and to increase services to existing groups. It will also present risks to be managed, by means of rigorous observation of standards for training, delegation, monitoring and supervision.

A further trend in workforce patterns is seen in the importance attributed to interprofessional working. The workshop participants identified this in the form of concern about multidisciplinary student placements. This concern may reflect either awareness of the potentially increased burden on SLTs asked to provide clinical education and support for students from diverse disciplines or fear that SLT student participation in multidisciplinary placements might dilute development of specific speech and language therapy skills.

Ethical issues in private practice, which has grown significantly in some countries as public services shrink or cannot keep pace with demand (American Speech-Language-Hearing Association [ASHA], (2008c); Lambier & Atherton, 2003), were a major topic of discussion in the workshop. As noted in Chapter 8, issues related to SLTs in private enterprise form the bulk of complaints to ethics boards in the USA and Australia. Some of these complaints relate to business practices, others to the provision of outdated or inappropriate services. Currency of knowledge and skills and fitness for practice are therefore key issues.

Fitness for practice has become a major focus of regulatory procedures in the profession in recent years. Limited opportunity or failure to take personal responsibility for accessing continuing professional development (CPD) (also sometimes termed learning beyond registration) were noted by workshop participants as ethical issues which would grow in importance over time as evidence-based practice is increasingly demanded by consumers, managers and reimbursement agencies. Participation in CPD can be problematic for private practitioners, who typically have to pay for their professional development despite loss of work time and income. However, it is also a problem for SLTs in public employment, where employers may provide little or no financial support for CPD, or may not make backfill available to allow SLTs to attend CPD events. For rural and remote SLTs the time and cost involved in travel to and from CPD events make participation even more challenging.

Service users and service delivery

Failure to keep abreast of theoretical and practical progress in the field of communication and swallowing impairment is likely to become increasingly exposed in the face of growing health consumerism on the part of service users. As the internet becomes more widely available in homes, clients and their families will become more sophisticated consumers of healthcare information and services, as Scenario 7.2 illustrated. Well-informed consumers will have high expectations of best practice and efficient and accessible healthcare service delivery. They are also likely to recognise value for money more easily when they are paying for private services. The growing sophistication of healthcare consumers in terms of knowledge and expectations will have implications for the way in which SLTs manage ethically sensitive tasks like disclosure of information.

Consumers' demands for services delivered in or closer to their home are likely to prompt increasing use of telehealth. The field is already in development, with studies reported of therapy for voice disorders (Mashima et al., 2003), motor speech disorders (Hill et al., 2006) and stuttering (C. Lewis, Packman, Onslow, Simpson & Jones, 2008), for example. The field covers a range of technologies, from telephones to videoconferencing and internet-based systems, and a variety of technological challenges will need to be overcome (Theodoros, 2008). Although services delivered into people's homes represent a promising development for adults and children with a range of impairments, this mode of service delivery will not be without ethical and legal risks. According to a report prepared for ASHA (2001), 'telepractice will present major ethical challenges to the unwary' (p. 8). In fact, it is equally likely to present challenges to the wary. A recent special edition of the *Cambridge Quarterly of Healthcare Ethics* has described the ethical landscape of electronic healthcare as the 'newest frontier', an ethical landscape that might represent anything from 'a technologic garden of healthcare delights' to 'a technological abyss where patients and health professionals are alienated from each other' (Bauer, 2008, p. 358).

Access to telehealth constitutes a major logistical and ethically pressing challenge. The concept of 'meaningful access' encompasses the fact that even if users have necessary funds to purchase relevant equipment, they 'may not have the skills or resources they need to use technology, diagnose and solve technical problems, afford continuous service charges, or locate and understand content' (Baur, 2008, p. 418). Unfortunately, as Baur further states, 'the same population groups that have poorer health status also have less access to the internet and health information' (p. 417). Thus, a central ethical question regarding telehealth is whether its development will actually serve to exacerbate already existing health inequalities.

Privacy and confidentiality are not particularly easy to maintain in the course of direct therapy interactions and associated care. The complexities of internet and telecommunications security are likely to make this challenge greater. In addition, as more health information about individuals is held electronically, issues of incorrect and obsolete data will need to be addressed. Protocols for access to electronic data or transmissions will need to be sufficiently clear for participants in telehealth projects to give consent that is properly informed.

We have argued throughout this book that the nature of relationships that SLTs have with the people who use their services is central to the ethical quality of the work. It will therefore be important to monitor and evaluate the quality of human interactions conducted at a distance. It may be, for example, that telehealth applications are perceived as impersonal and create a greater sense of isolation (Cornford & Klecun-Dabrowska, 2001). On the other hand, we need to bear in mind that telehealth applications appear to have enormous potential to extend services to people who might not otherwise have access and to be a force for empowerment of service users and for democratisation of health.

Ethics education

It is now generally acknowledged that teaching of ethics should form part of speech and language therapy education. In Australia, for example, the standards (Speech Pathology Australia, 2001) which govern practice and accreditation of speech and language therapy courses make it clear that ethics education is an expected part of the curriculum. In this final section of our book we consider the issue of ethics education for current and future SLTs and methods for delivering it.

Ethics education for clinicians and students might be seen as a way of potentially decreasing the need for regulation and remedial action by statutory bodies in response to complaints. As Pannbacker (2005), notes, it is clearly 'preferable to strengthen speech-language pathologists' ethical awareness and clinical practice by education rather than denunciation' (p. 19), a view with which it is difficult to disagree. Raising ethical awareness across the board is an approach strongly advocated by McAllister (2005). This approach avoids a language of 'dilemmas' and even of ethics being solely about decision making, and instead focuses on raising awareness of the ethical dimensions to everything we do and say in our daily practice. The difference between the two approaches to ethics is considerable: regulation is primarily reactive and in essence punitive, dealing only with problems once reported; the alternative is proactive and aspirational, conceptualising ethics as being about more than just problems. This takes us back to the discussion in Chapter 1 about the nature and importance of ethics and about its place at 'the heart of healthcare', to borrow from the title of a book by Seedhouse (2005). In this conceptualisation, ethics education is about encouraging people to develop the practice of considering the purpose of what it is they are doing and the manner in which they are trying to achieve that purpose.

The inclusion of ethics teaching in pre-qualification curricula is not necessarily straightforward. Irwin et al. (2007), in a supplementary instructor's manual to their book on ethics, acknowledge that it is not a subject area in which many academics specialise and that its complexities can make it a daunting area for non-specialists to teach (hence the manual provided by Irwin et al. as an aid to teaching). Similar arguments, however, are likely to apply to other developing subject areas, such as telehealth discussed above. Academic curricula are in a state of constant development. Fitting ethics teaching into a curriculum can be equally as challenging as finding people to teach it, especially in contest with direct clinical teaching. Students might be forgiven for seeing ethics teaching as a waste of their limited time. Our view would be that leaving ethics out of education is akin to building a wall with lots of bricks and no mortar. Ethics is what keeps the whole endeavour together and potentially makes it strong.

Once ethics has a place in the curriculum, how should we teach it? There are some formal published packages for teaching ethics in speech and language therapy, such as those by Chabon, Denton, Lansing, Scudder and Shinn (2007) and the previously mentioned instructor's manual from Irwin et al. (2007). These favour a programmed approach to ethics, basing the teaching on the principles and rules found in the Code of Ethics of ASHA. The approach to ethics we have taken in this book is rather more pluralistic.

As we noted in Chapter 2, by far the most common approach to ethics education in the healthcare professions is based on the principles outlined by Beauchamp and Childress (2005) and the various decision-making protocols that have grown out of them. As we have discussed, there are a number of other biomedically derived systems. The four quadrants (Jonsen et al., 1982; Sokol, 2008) approach advocates starting with the (medical) problem itself and zooming out to the wider social perspective. The CARE approach (Schneider & Snell, 2000) proposes tackling ethical problems by considering *c*ore beliefs, *a*ctions, *r*easons and *e*xperience (hence the acronym). Although it is certainly important for students and clinicians to know the basics of these different approaches, they all deal with ethics fundamentally as a sequence of dilemmas to be dealt with. In addition, the linearity of most protocols obscures the complex iterative and unfolding nature of the ethical issues at hand.

Students in clinical practice tend to have relatively little experience of outright ethical dilemmas. What they do have in abundance, though, is experience of people and of interactions with them. This suggests that alternative ways of thinking about ethics may be at least as important as principles and protocols. We have already discussed the ethics of care (Chapter 2) and its focus on the relationship between care giver and care receiver. Since students and teachers are familiar not only with people and interactions but also with stories about people, narrative ethics (Charon, 2006; Charon & Montello, 2002) is another way of thinking about ethics in healthcare that is worthy of consideration. Discussing narratives about people and interactions, or, as we referred to it at the start of this chapter, talking it through, may assist tellers to resolve a problem or to consider why they have had a particular interaction with someone; it may also raise ethical awareness in others engaged in the discussion. We have endeavoured to exemplify ethical thinking by means of narratives throughout the book.

The complexity of interrelated and possibly conflicting perspectives of the multiple players in most situations encountered in allied health and social care practice makes narrative ethics an appealing alternative or adjunct to decision-making protocols founded on biomedical principles. As Kirschner et al. (2001) report, allied health professionals favour discussion as the best way of learning and thinking about ethics. Narrative approaches to ethics allow insights into the concerns and motivations of the multiple players in any situation, and such approaches may better prepare students for the lack of consensus they will inevitably encounter in current healthcare practice and in dealing with emerging ethical trends as outlined above. They might also help students conceptualise ethics as less about problems and more about people. Charon and Montello (2002, p. xi) provide a useful insight into ethics from the perspective of patients in the introduction to their book on narrative ethics:

> The ethics under question are not located primarily in the technical questions of providing or withholding health care, allocating scarce resources, or preserving autonomy in the face of death. Those are ethicists' ethical considerations. In large part, the ethics in question are the ethics of ordinary life: how to fulfil goals, to honor obligations, and to make sense of events in ways that make it possible to go on. (p. xi)

Finally, it is important to recognise that learning about ethics does not stop at the time of qualification. The ultimate purpose of this book has been to prompt more discussion of all aspects of ethics within speech and language therapy as a whole. The book is intended as just one contribution to that ongoing discussion.

A final thought

We finish the book by returning to the therapy interaction between one of the authors (RB) and Mrs Davies. In Chapter 1 we described the subtlety surrounding the use of the seemingly innocuous word 'yet'. Mrs Davies, from whom I learned an awful lot, also presented me with another significant ethical challenge.

In her medical notes was written, in red ink, the instruction: 'Daughter does not want patient to know diagnosis.' The diagnosis, you may recall, was motor neurone disease. I did have the awareness to query this position with the medical staff and was advised about a suitable response. 'Tell her she's got a muscle-wasting disease that might get better.' With hindsight this was, of course, an entirely unsuitable response. It would be nice to think that this situation does not arise these days. Sadly, I did not have the clinical wherewithal at that time to think through the implications of this advice, strange as that feels to admit now. In circumstances similar to those surrounding the conversation involving 'yet' – in her front room on a hot, airless afternoon – she asked me, 'Do I have motor neurone disease?' I did not use the response that had been suggested. We would like to leave readers to consider how this question could have best been answered.

References

Adshead, G. (2002). A different voice in psychiatric ethics. In K. Fulford, D. Dickenson & T. Murray (Eds.), *Healthcare ethics and human values* (pp. 56–62). Oxford: Blackwell.

Allmark, P. (2002). Can there be an ethics of care? In K. Fulford, D. Dickenson & T. Murray (Eds.), *Healthcare ethics and human values* (pp. 63–69). Oxford: Blackwell.

Almost, D., & Rosenbaum, P. (1998). Effectiveness of speech intervention for phonological disorders: A randomized controlled trial. *Developmental Medicine and Child Neurology, 40*, 319–325.

Alzheimer's Society. (2008). What is dementia? Retrieved August 18, 2008 from www.alzheimers.org.uk

American Speech-Language-Hearing Association. (1990). Prevention of communication disorders. *ASHA, 33*, 15–41.

American Speech-Language-Hearing Association. (1992). Instrumental diagnostic procedures for swallowing. *ASHA, 34*, 25–33.

American Speech-Language-Hearing Association. (2001). *Telepractices and ASHA: Report of the telepractices team*. Rockville, MD: ASHA.

American Speech-Language-Hearing Association. (2003). *Code of ethics*. Rockville, MD: ASHA.

American Speech-Language-Hearing Association. (2004). Guidelines for the training, use, and supervision of speech-language pathology assistants. Retrieved September 25, 2008 from www.asha.org/policy

American Speech-Language-Hearing Association. (2005). Cultural competence. Retrieved September 25, 2008 from www.asha.org/policy

American Speech-Language-Hearing Association. (2007). Membership profile: Highlights and trends. Retrieved September 25, 2008 from www.asha.org/about/membership-certification/member-counts.htm

American Speech-Language-Hearing Association. (2008a). Accepting referrals for private practice from primary place of employment. Retrieved September 25, 2008 from www.asha.org/policy.

American Speech-Language-Hearing Association. (2008b). Client abandonment. Retrieved September 25, 2008 from www.asha.org/policy

American Speech-Language-Hearing Association. (2008c). How we've changed: ASHA members and affiliates in private practice, 1996 and 2006. Retrieved September 25, 2008 from www.asha.org/NR/rdonlyres/BC8F5071-578F-4C71-8756-2B7B979AF573/0/06HWCprivatepractice.pdf

American Speech-Language-Hearing Association. (2008d). Incidence and prevalence of speech, voice, and language disorders in adults in the United States: 2008 edition. Retrieved September 25, 2008 from www.asha.org/members/research/reports/speech_voice_language.htm.

Antaki, C. (2001). 'D'you like a drink then do you?' Dissembling language and the construction of an impoverished life. *Journal of Language and Social Psychology, 20,* 196–213.

Armstrong, E. (2003). Communication culture in acute speech pathology settings: Current issues. *Advances in Speech-Language Pathology, 5,* 137–143.

Arnesen, T., & Nord, E. (1999). The value of DALY life: Problems with ethics and validity of disability adjusted life years. *British Medical Journal, 319,* 1423–1425.

Baines, P. (2008). Medical ethics for children: Applying the four principles to paediatrics. *Journal of Medical Ethics, 34,* 141–145.

Balandin, S., & Lincoln, M. (2003). Swallowing and communication: Are we eating our words? *Advances in Speech-Language Pathology, 5,* 119–124.

Battle, D. (Ed.). (2002). *Communication disorders in multicultural populations* (3rd ed.). New York: Butterworth-Heinemann.

Bauer, K. (2008). Guest editorial. *Cambridge Quarterly of Healthcare Ethics, 17,* 358–359.

Baur, C. (2008). An analysis of factors underlying e-health disparities. *Cambridge Quarterly of Healthcare Ethics, 17,* 417–428.

Beauchamp, T., & Childress, J. (2009). *Principles of biomedical ethics* (6th ed).. Oxford: Oxford University Press.

Belenky, M., Clinchy, B., Goldberger, N., & Tarule, J. (1997). *Women's ways of knowing: The development of self, voice and mind.* New York: Basic Books.

Benjamin, A. (2008, May 14). Written in the stars. *The Guardian: Society,* p. 7.

Berglund, C. (2007). *Ethics for health care* (3rd ed.). South Melbourne: Oxford University Press.

Beukelman, D., & Mirenda, P. (2005). *Augmentative and alternative communication: Supporting children and adults with complex communication needs* (3rd ed.). Baltimore: Paul H. Brookes.

Blackhall, L., Murphy, S., Frank, G., Michel, V., & Azen, S. (1995). Ethnicity and attitudes towards patient autonomy. *Journal of the American Medical Association, 274,* 820–825.

Blake, H. (2008). Caregiver stress in traumatic brain injury. *International Journal of Therapy and Rehabilitation, 15,* 263–271.

Body, R., & Perkins, M. (2006). Terminology and methodology in the assessment of cognitive-linguistic ability after traumatic brain injury. *Brain Impairment, 7,* 212–222.

Boon, H., Verhoef, M., O'Hara, D., & Findlay, B. (2004). From parallel practice to integrative health care: A conceptual framework. *BMC Health Services Research, 4,* 1–5.

Boyle, J., McCartney, E., Forbes, J., & O'Hare, A. (2007). A randomised controlled trial and economic evaluation of direct versus indirect and individual versus group modes of speech and language therapy for children with primary language impairment. *Health Technology and Assessment, 11,* 1–139.

Brannelly, T. (2006). Negotiating ethics in dementia care: An analysis of an ethic of care in practice. *Dementia, 5*, 197–212.

Braunack-Mayer, J. (2001). What makes a problem an ethical problem? An ethical perspective on the nature of ethical problems in general practice. *Journal of Medical Ethics, 27*, 98–103.

Braveman, P., & Gruskin, S. (2003). Poverty, equity, human rights and health. *World Health Organization Bulletin, 81*, 539–545.

Brenner, P. (1997). A dialogue between virtue ethics and care ethics. *Theoretical Medicine and Bioethics, 18*, 47–61.

Brody, H. (2002). 'My story is broken; Can you help me fix it?' Medical ethics and the joint construction of narrative. In K. Fulford, D. Dickenson & T. Murray (Eds.), *Healthcare ethics and human values* (pp. 133–140). Oxford: Blackwell.

Bronfenbrenner, U. (1994). Ecological models of human development. In T. Husen & T. Postlethwaite (Eds.), *International encyclopaedia of education* (2nd ed., pp. 1643–1647). Oxford: Pergamon Press.

Broomfield, J., & Dodd, B. (2004). Children with speech and language disability: Caseload characteristics. *International Journal of Language and Communication Disorders*, 303–324.

Browne, A., & Browne, K. (2007). Morality, prudential rationality, and cheating. *Cambridge Quarterly of Healthcare Ethics, 16*, 53–62.

Brumfitt, S., Atkinson, J., & Greated, G. (1994). The carer's response to written information about acquired communication problems. *Aphasiology, 8*, 583–590.

Bryan, K. (2004). Preliminary study of the prevalence of speech and language difficulties in young offenders. *International Journal of Language and Communication Disorders, 39*, 391–400.

Byng, S., Cairns, D., & Duchan, J. (2002). Values in practice and practising values. *Journal of Communication Disorders, 35*, 89–106.

Byng, S., Kay, J., Edmundson, A., & Scott, C. (1990). Aphasia tests reconsidered. *Aphasiology, 4*, 67–91.

Campbell, A., Gillett, G., & Jones, G. (2001). *Medical ethics* (3rd ed.). Oxford: Oxford University Press.

Campbell, T. (1999). Functional treatment outcomes in young children with motor speech disorders. In A. Caruso & E. Strand (Eds.), *Clinical management of motor speech disorders in children* (pp. 385–396). New York: Thieme Medical.

Canadian Association of Speech-Language Pathologists and Audiologists. (2005). *Code of ethics*. Ottawa: Canadian Association of Speech-Language Pathologists and Audiologists.

Carey, P. (2006). *Theft: A love story*. London: Faber and Faber.

Centers for Disease Control. (2008). Facts about traumatic brain injury. Retrieved August 18, 2008 from www.cdc.gov/ncipc/tbi/FactSheets/Facts_About_TBI.pdf

Chabon, S., Denton, D., Lansing, C., Scudder, R., & Shinn, R. (2007). *Ethics education*. Rockville, MD: American Speech-Language-Hearing Association.

Chabon, S., & Morris, J. (2004, February 17). A consensus model for making ethical decisions in a less-than-ideal-world. *The ASHA Leader, 9*(3), 18–19.

Chabon, S., & Ulrich, S. (2006, February 7). Uses and abuses of the ASHA Code of Ethics. *The ASHA Leader, 11*(2), 22–23.

Charon, R. (2006). *Narrative medicine: Honoring the stories of illness*. Oxford: Oxford University Press.

Charon, R., & Montello, M. (Eds.). (2002). *Stories matter: The role of narrative in medical ethics*. London: Routledge.

Cheng, L. (2000). Children of yesterday, today and tomorrow: Global implications for child language. *Phoniatrica et Logopaedica, 52*, 39–47.

Christiansen, J., & Leigh, I. (2002). *Cochlear implants in children: Ethics and choices*. Washington, DC: Gallaudet University Press.

Christiansen, J., & Leigh, I. (2004). Changing parent and deaf community perspectives. *Archives of Otolaryngology – Head and Neck Surgery, 130*, 673–677.

Clark, H. (1996). *Using language*. Cambridge: Cambridge University Press.

Cockburn, T. (2005). Children and the feminist ethic of care. *Childhood, 12*, 71–89.

Colicutt McGrath, J. (2007). *Ethical practice in brain injury rehabilitation*. Oxford: Oxford University Press.

Conlin, K., Mirus, G., Mauk, C., & Meier, R. (2000). The acquisition of first signs: Place, handshape, and movement. In C. Chamberlain, J. Morford & R. Mayberry (Eds.), *Language acquisition by eye* (pp. 51–70). Mahwah, NJ: Erlbaum.

Cook, J. (1980). The delegation of surgical responsibility. *Journal of Medical Ethics, 6*, 68–70.

Cornford, T., & Klecun-Dabrowska, E. (2001). Ethical perspectives in evaluation of telehealth. *Cambridge Quarterly of Healthcare Ethics, 10*, 161–169.

Cott, C. (1998). Structure and meaning in multidisciplinary teamwork. *Sociology of Health and Illness, 20*, 848–873.

Cowley, C. (2005). The dangers of medical ethics. *Journal of Medical Ethics, 31*, 739–742.

Crary, M., & Groher, M. (2003). *Introduction to adult swallowing disorders*. Philadelphia: Butterworth-Heinemann.

Cribb, A., & Duncan, P. (2002). *Health promotion and professional ethics*. Oxford: Blackwell.

Cross, E., Goodacres, S., & O'Chathain, A. (2006). Rationing in the emergency department: The good, the bad, and the unacceptable. *Emergency Medicine Journal, 22*, 171–176.

Cross, R., Leitão, S., & McAllister, L. (2008). Think big, act locally: Responding to ethical dilemmas. *ACQuiring Knowledge in Speech, Language and Hearing, 10*, 39–41.

Cruice, M. (2007). Issues of inclusion and access with aphasia. *Aphasiology, 21*, 3–8.

Cull, A., Miller, H., Porterfield, T., Mackay, J., Anderson, E., Steel, C., et al. (1998). The use of videotaped information in cancer genetic counselling: A randomized evaluation study. *British Journal of Cancer, 77*, 830–837.

Daniels, N. (1985). *Just health care*. Cambridge: Cambridge University Press.

de Koning, H., de Ridder-Sluiter, J., van Agt, H., Reep-van den Bergh, C., van der Stege, H., Korfage, I., et al. (2004). A cluster-randomised trial of screening for language disorders in toddlers. *Journal of Medical Screening, 11*, 109–116.

Department for Children, Schools and Families. (2008). *A review of services for children and young people (0–19) with speech, language and communication needs*. London: Department for Children, Schools and Families.

Department for Education and Employment. (1999). *Sure Start: A guide for second wave programmes*. London: Department for Education and Employment.

Department for Education and Skills. (1999). *Sure Start: A guide for trailblazers*. London: Department for Education and Skills.

Department of Health. (2003). The Chief Health Professions Officer's ten key roles for allied health professionals. Retrieved July 8, 2008 from www.dh.gov.uk/assetRoot/04/06/16/12/04061612.pdf

Donnellan, A. (1984). The criterion of the least dangerous assumption. *Behavioral Disorders, 9*, 141–150.

Downie, R., & Macnaughton, J. (2007). *Bioethics and the humanities: Attitudes and perceptions*. Abingdon: Routledge Cavendish.

Drew, P. (2006). Misalignments in 'after-hours' calls to a British GP practice: A study in telephone medicine. In J. Heritage & D. Maynard (Eds.), *Communication in medical care: Interaction between primary care physicians and patients* (pp. 416–444). Cambridge: Cambridge University Press.

Duchan, J., Calculator, S., Sonnenmeier, R., Diehl, S., & Cumley, G. (2001). A framework for managing controversial practices. *Language, Speech, and Hearing Services in Schools, 32*, 133–141.

Duchan, J., Maxwell, M., & Kovarsky, D. (1999). Evaluating competence in the course of everyday interactions. In D. Kovarsky, J. Duchan & M. Maxwell (Eds.), *Constructing (in)competence: Disabling valuations in clinical and social interaction* (pp. 3–26). Mahwah, NJ: Erlbaum.

Duffy, J. (2005). *Motor speech disorders: Substrates, differential diagnosis, and management* (2nd ed.). St. Louis: Elsevier Mosby.

Duncan, D., White, J., & Nicholson, T. (2003). Using internet-based surveys to reach hidden populations: Case of nonabusive illicit drug users. *American Journal of Health Behavior, 27*, 208–218.

Dunst, C., Trivette, C., & Deal, A. (1994). *Supporting and strengthening families: Methods, strategies and practices*. Cambridge, MA: Brookline.

Edwards, D. (2006). Facts, norms and dispositions: Practical uses of the modal verb 'would' in police interrogations. *Discourse Studies, 8*, 475–501.

Egan, C. (1990). *The skilled helper: A systematic approach to effective helping*. Pacific Grove, CA: Brooks/Cole.

Ehlers, S., & Gillberg, C. (1993). The epidemiology of Asperger syndrome: A total population study. *Journal of Child Psychology and Psychiatry, 34*, 1327–1350.

Enderby, P., & Petheram, B. (2002). Has aphasia therapy been swallowed up? *Clinical Rehabilitation, 16*, 604–608.

Epstein-Frisch, B., van Dam, T., & Chenoweth, L. (2006). *Presenting the evidence: Accommodation and support for people with disability*. Epping, NSW: Institute for Family Advocacy and Leadership Development.

Felsenfeld, S., Broen, P., & McGue, M. (1992). A 28-year follow-up of adults with a history of moderate phonological disorder: Linguistic and personality results. *Journal of Speech and Hearing Research, 35*, 1114–1125.

Felsenfeld, S., Broen, P., & McGue, M. (1994). A 28-year follow-up of adults with a history of moderate phonological disorder: Educational and occupational results. *Journal of Speech and Hearing Research, 37*, 1341–1353.

Ferguson, K. (2005). Professional supervision. In M. Rose & D. Best (Eds.), *Transforming practice through clinical education, professional supervision and mentoring* (pp. 293–307). Edinburgh: Elsevier.

Finlay, W., Antaki, C., & Walton, C. (2008). Saying no to the staff: An analysis of refusals in a home for people with severe communication difficulties. *Sociology of Health and Illness, 30*, 55–75.

Fisher, C. (2003). *Decoding the ethics code*. Thousand Oaks, CA: Sage.

Folkins, J. (1992). Resource on person-first language. Retrieved August 13, 2008 from http://www.asha.org/about/publications/journal-abstracts/submissions/person_first.htm#1

Freeman, J. (2006). Ethical theory and medical ethics: A personal perspective. *Journal of Medical Ethics, 32*, 617–618.

Fujiki, M., Brinton, B., Isaacson, T., & Summers, C. (2001). Social behaviors of children with language impairment on the playground: A pilot study. *Language, Speech, and Hearing Services in Schools, 32*, 101–113.

Fulford, K., Dickenson, D., & Murray, T. (2002). Many voices: Human values in healthcare ethics. In K. Fulford, D. Dickenson & T. Murray (Eds.), *Healthcare ethics and human values* (pp. 1–19). Oxford: Blackwell.

Fulford, K., & Hope, R. (1993). Psychiatric ethics: A bioethical ugly duckling? In R. Gillon & A. Lloyd (Eds.), *Principles of health care ethics* (pp. 681–695). Chichester: Wiley.

Gardiner, P. (2003). A virtue ethics approach to moral dilemmas in medicine. *Journal of Medical Ethics, 2*, 297–302.

Gardner, H. (2006). Training others in the art of therapy for speech sound disorders: An interactional approach. *Child Language Teaching and Therapy, 22*, 27–46.

Gillam, S., & Gillam, R. (2006). Making evidence-based decisions about child language intervention in schools. *Language, Speech, and Hearing Services in Schools, 37*, 304–315.

Gilligan, C. (1982). *In a different voice: Psychological theory and women's development*. Cambridge, MA: Harvard University Press.

Gillon, R. (2003). Ethics needs principles – four can encompass the rest – and respect for autonomy should be 'first among equals'. *Journal of Medical Ethics, 29*, 307–312.

Glogowska, M., Roulstone, S., Enderby, P., & Peters, T. (2000). Randomised controlled trial of community based speech and language therapy in preschool children. *British Medical Journal, 321*, 923–926.

Grove, N., & Walker, M. (1990). The Makaton vocabulary: Using manual signs and graphic symbols to develop interpersonal communication. *Augmentative and Alternative Communication, 6*, 15–28.

Gutman, V. (2005). Ethical reasoning and mental health services with deaf clients. *Journal of Deaf Studies and Deaf Education, 10*, 171–183.

Hack, M. (2007). Survival and neurodevelopmental outcomes of preterm infants. *Journal of Pediatric Gastroenterology and Nutrition, 45*(Suppl. 3), S141–S142.

Hagen, C. (1982). Language-cognitive disorganization following closed head injury: A conceptualization. In L. Trexler (Ed.), *Cognitive rehabilitation: Conceptualization and intervention* (pp. 131–149). New York: Plenum Press.

Halliday, M., & Hasan, R. (1985). *Language, context, and text: Aspects of language in a social-semiotic perspective.* Waurn Ponds, Vic.: Deakin University.

Hammer, C. (1998). Toward a 'thick description' of families: Using ethnography to overcome the obstacles to providing family-centered early intervention services. *American Journal of Speech-Language Pathology, 7*, 5–22.

Hand, L. (2006). Clinicians as 'information givers': What communication access are clients given to speech-language pathology services? *Topics in Language Disorders, 26*, 240–265.

Hansson, S. (2005). Implant ethics. *Journal of Medical Ethics, 31*, 519–525.

Harris, J. (2003). In praise of unprincipled ethics. *Journal of Medical Ethics, 29*, 303–308.

Health Professions Council. (2008). *Standards of conduct, performance and ethics.* London: Health Professions Council.

Hendrick, J. (2000). *Law and ethics in nursing and health care.* Oxford: Stanley Thornes.

Hersh, D. (2002). *Ethics and treatment termination: Speech pathologists' views of ending aphasia therapy.* Paper presented at the Australian Bioethics Association Conference, Adelaide.

Hersh, D. (2003). 'Weaning' clients from aphasia therapy: Speech pathologists' strategies for discharge. *Aphasiology, 17*, 1007–1029.

Hill, A., Theodoros, D., Russell, T., Cahill, L., Ward, E., & Clark, K. (2006). An internet-based telerehabilitation system for the assessment of motor speech disorders: A pilot study. *American Journal of Speech-Language Pathology, 15*, 45–56.

Horner Catt, J. (2000). The language of ethics in clinical practice. *Journal of Medical Speech-Language Pathology, 8*, 137–153.

Horton, S. (2008). Learning-in-interaction: Resourceful work by people with aphasia and therapists in the course of language impairment therapy. *Aphasiology, 22*, 985–1014.

Hyde, M., & Power, D. (2006). Some ethical dimensions of cochlear implantation for deaf children and their families. *Journal of Deaf Studies and Deaf Education, 11*, 102–111.

Irwin, D., Pannbacker, M., Powell, T., & Vekovius, G. (2007). *Ethics for speech-language pathologists and audiologists: An illustrative casebook.* New York: Delmar.

Isaac, K. (2002). *Speech pathology in cultural and linguistic diversity.* London: Whurr.

Jones, B., Clark, G., & Stolz, D. (1997). Characteristics and practices of sign language interpreters in inclusive education programs. *Exceptional Children, 63*, 257–268.

Jones, M., Onslow, M., Packman, A., Williams, S., Ormond, T., Schwarz, I., et al. (2005). Randomised controlled trial of the Lidcombe programme of early stuttering intervention. *British Medical Journal, 331*, 659–663.

Jones, T. (1991). Ethical decision making by individuals in organizations: An issue-contingent model. *Academy of Management Review, 16*, 366–395.

Jonsen, A., Siegler, M., & Winslade, W. (1982). *Clinical ethics.* New York: McGraw-Hill.

Jorgensen, C., McSheehan, M., & Sonnenmeier, R. (2007). Presumed competence reflected in educational programs of students with IDD before and after the Beyond Access professional development intervention. *Journal of Intellectual and Developmental Disabilities, 32*, 238–262.

Kadushin, A. (1968). Games people play in supervision. *Social Work, 18*, 23–32.

Kagan, A., Black, S., Duchan, J., Simmons-Mackie, N., & Square, S. (2001). Training volunteers as conversation partners using 'Supported Conversation for Adults with Aphasia' (SCA). *Journal of Speech, Language, and Hearing Research, 44*, 624–638.

Kenny, B., Lincoln, N., & Balandin, S. (2007). A dynamic model of ethical reasoning in speech pathology. *Journal of Medical Ethics*, *38*, 508–513.

Kind, A., Smith, M., Frytak, J., & Finch, M. (2007). Bouncing back: Patterns and predictors of complicated transitions 30 days after hospitalization for acute ischemic stroke. *Journal of the American Geriatrics Society*, *55*, 365–373.

Kinsella, E. A. (2005). Constructions of self: Ethical overtones in surprising locations. *Medical Humanities*, *31*, 67–71.

Kirschner, K., Stocking, C., Wagner, L., Foye, S., & Siegler, M. (2001). Ethical issues identified by rehabilitation clinicians. *Archives of Physical Medicine and Rehabilitation*, *82*(Suppl. 2), S2–S8.

Knox, E., & Conti-Ramsden, G. (2003). Bullying risks of 11-year-old children with specific language impairment (SLI): Does school placement matter? *International Journal of Language and Communication Disorders*, *38*, 1–12.

Kornfeld, J., Fleisher, L., Maat, J., Vanchieri, C., Hohenemser, L., & Stevens, N. (1998). Reaching minority and underserved populations: The impact of the cancer information service's outreach program. Part 3. *Journal of Health Communication*, *3*, 36–49.

Kovarsky, D., Duchan, J., & Maxwell, M. (Eds.). (1999). *Constructing (in)competence: Disabling evaluations in clinical and social interaction*. Mahwah, NJ: Erlbaum.

Lambier, J., & Atherton, M. (2003). *General membership survey*. Melbourne: Speech Pathology Australia.

Lamont, S., & Brown, L. (2001). *The jury is out: Ethical issues in allied health care*: Workshop presented at the 4th National Allied Health Conference, Fremantle, Western Australia.

Landes, T. (1999). Ethical issues involved in patients' rights to refuse artificially administered nutrition and hydration and implications for the speech-language pathologist. *American Journal of Speech-Language Pathology*, *8*, 109–117.

Lane, H., & Bahan, B. (1998). Ethics of cochlear implantation in young children: A review and reply from a Deaf-World perspective. *Otolaryngology – Head and Neck Surgery*, *119*, 297–313.

Lane, H., & Grodin, M. (1997). Ethical issues in cochlear implant surgery: An exploration into disease, disability, and the best interests of the child. *Kennedy Institute of Ethics Journal*, *7*, 231–251.

Langmore, S., Skarupski, K., Park, P., & Fries, B. (2002). Predictors of aspiration pneumonia in nursing home residents. *Dysphagia*, *17*, 298–307.

Langmore, S., Terpenning, M., Schork, A., Chen, Y., Murray, J., Lopatin, D., et al. (2001). Predictors of aspiration pneumonia: How important is dysphagia? *Dysphagia*, *13*, 69–81.

Law, J., Boyle, J., Harris, F., Harkness, A., & Nye, C. (1998). Screening for speech and language delay: A systematic review of the literature. *Health Technology and Assessment*, *2*, 1–185.

Law, J., Boyle, J., Harris, F., Harkness, A., & Nye, C. (2000). Prevalence and natural history of primary speech and language delay: Findings from a systematic review of the literature. *International Journal of Language and Communication Disorders*, *35*, 165–188.

Law, J., Garrett, Z., & Nye, C. (2003). Speech and language therapy interventions for children with primary speech and language delay or disorder. *Cochrane Database of Systematic Review*, *3*, CD004110.

Lawrence, R., & Curlin, F. (2007). Clash of definitions: Controversies about conscience in medicine. *American Journal of Bioethics*, *7*, 10–14.

Lees, J. (2005). *Children with acquired aphasias* (2nd ed). Chichester: Wiley.

Levy, N. (2002). Reconsidering cohclear implants: The lessons of Martha's Vineyard. *Bioethics, 16*, 134–153.

Lewis, C., Packman, A., Onslow, M., Simpson, J., & Jones, M. (2008). A phase II trial of telehealth delivery of the Lidcombe program of early stuttering intervention. *American Journal of Speech-Language Pathology, 17*, 139–149.

Lewis, J. (2002). Doctor. In K. Fulford, D. Dickenson & J. Murray (Eds.), *Healthcare ethics and human values* (p. 166). Oxford: Blackwell.

Lobb, E., Butow, P., Barratt, A., Meiser, B., Gaff, C., Young, M., et al. (2004). Communication and information-giving in high-risk breast cancer consultations: Influence on patient outcomes. *British Journal of Cancer, 90*, 321–327.

Lock, S., & Wilkinson, R. (2001). Supporting partners of people with aphasia in relationships and conversation (SPPARC). *International Journal of Language and Communication Disorders, 36*(Suppl.), 25–30.

Logemann, J. (1998). *Evaluation and treatment of swallowing disorders* (2nd ed.). Austin, TX: Pro-Ed.

Mackey, H. (2005). Assistant practitioners: Issues of accountability, delegation and competence. *International Journal of Therapy and Rehabilitation, 12*, 331–338.

Macklin, R. (1999). *Against relativism*. New York: Oxford University Press.

Malec, J. (1993). Ethics in brain injury rehabilitation: Existential choices among Western cultural beliefs. *Brain Injury, 7*, 383–400.

Malloy, D., Williams, J., Hadjistavropoulos, T., Krishnan, B., Jeyaraj, M., McCarthy, E., et al. (2006). Ethical decision-making about older adults and moral intensity: An international study of physicians. *Journal of Medical Ethics, 34*, 285–296.

Mansell, J. (2006). Deinstitutionalisation and community living: Progress, problems and priorities. *Journal of Intellectual and Developmental Disabilities, 31*, 65–76.

Marcus, G., & Fisher, S. (2003). *FOXP2* in focus: What can genes tell us about speech and language? *Trends in Cognitive Sciences, 7*, 257–262.

Martino, R., Beaton, D., & Diamant, N. (in press). Using different perspectives to generate items for a new scale measuring medical outcomes of dysphagia (MOD). *Journal of Clinical Epidemiology.*

Mashima, P., Birkmire-Peters, D., Syms, M., Holtel, M., Burgess, L., & Peters, L. (2003). Telehealth: Voice therapy using telecommunications technology. *American Journal of Speech-Language Pathology, 12*, 432–439.

Mattson, C., Mårild, S., & Pehrsson, N. (2001). Evaluation of a language-screening programme for 2.5-year-olds at Child Health Centres in Sweden. *Acta Paediatrica, 90*, 339–344.

Mayeroff, M. (1971). *On caring*. New York: Harper & Row.

McAllister, L. (2006). Ethics in the workplace: More than just using ethical decision-making protocols. *ACQuiring Knowledge in Speech, Language and Hearing, 8*, 76–80.

McKie, J., & Richardson, J. (2003). The rule of rescue. *Social Science and Medicine, 56*, 2407–2419.

McLean, S., & Mason, J. (2003). *Legal and ethical aspects of healthcare*. London: Greenwich Medical Media.

Meaburn, E., Dale, P., Craig, I., & Plomin, R. (2002). Language-impaired children: No sign of the FOXP2 mutation. *NeuroReport, 13*, 1075–1077.

Metzger, M. (1999). *Sign language interpreting: Deconstructing the myth of neutrality.* Washington, DC: Gallaudet University Press.

Morris, K. (2001). Psychological distress in carers of head injured individuals: The provision of written information. *Brain Injury, 15*, 239–254.

Morton-Cooper, A., & Palmer, A. (2000). *Mentoring, preceptorship and clinical supervision: A guide to professional roles in clinical practice* (2nd ed.). Oxford: Blackwell.

Moster, D., Lie, R., & Markestad, T. (2008). Long-term medical and social consequences of preterm birth. *New England Journal of Medicine, 359*, 262–273.

Mount, B. (1992). *Person-centered planning: Finding directions for change using Personal Futures Planning.* New York: Graphic Futures.

Mount, B., & Zwernik, K. (1988). *It's never too early, it's never too late: A booklet about Personal Futures Planning.* Mears Park Centre, MN: Metropolitan Council.

National Association of the Deaf. (2000). Cochlear implants: NAD policy statement. Retrieved September 11, 2008 from www.nad.org/ciposition

Nelson, H., & Nelson, J. (1995). *The patient in the family: An ethics of medicine and families.* New York: Routledge.

Nelson, H., Nygren, P., Walker, M., & Panoscha, R. (2006). Screening for speech and language delay in preschool children: Systematic evidence review for the US preventive services task force. *Pediatrics, 117*, e298–e319.

New Zealand Speech-Language Therapists' Association. (2000). *Code of ethics.* Auckland: New Zealand Speech-Language Therapists' Association.

Nicholas, J., & Geers, A. (2007). Will they catch up? The role of age at cochlear implantation in the spoken language development of children with severe to profound hearing loss. *Journal of Speech, Language, and Hearing Research, 50*, 1048–1062.

Noddings, N. (1988). An ethic of caring and its implications for instructional arrangements. *American Journal of Education, 96*, 215–230.

Noddings, N. (2003). *Caring: A feminine approach to ethics and education* (2nd ed.). Berkeley: University of California Press.

Nord, E. (1995). The person-trade-off approach to valuing health care programs. *Medical Decision Making, 15*, 201–208.

Northern, J., & Downs, M. (2002). *Hearing in children* (5th ed.). Pennsylvania: Lipincott Williams & Wilkins.

Nunes, R. (2001). Ethical dimension of paediatric cochlear implantation. *Theoretical Medicine and Bioethics, 22*, 337–349.

Olson Wagner, C., Gray, L., & Potter, R. (1983). Communicative disorders in a group of adult female offenders. *Journal of Communication Disorders, 16*, 269–277.

Opie, A. (1997). Thinking teams thinking clients: Issues of discourse and representation in the work of health care teams. *Sociology of Health and Illness, 19*, 259–280.

Pannbacker, M. (1998). Whistleblowing in speech-language pathology. *American Journal of Speech-Language Pathology, 7*, 18–23.

Parker, M., & Dickenson, D. (2001). *The Cambridge medical ethics workbook.* Cambridge: Cambridge University Press.

Parsons, P. (2004). *Ethics in public relations: A guide to best practice*. London: Chartered Institute of Public Relations.

Paul, R. (2007). *Language disorders from infancy through adolescence* (3rd ed.). St. Louis: Mosby.

Pertile, J., & Page, F. (2003). The Maroondah Approach to Clinical Services (MACS): An integrated service delivery system. *ACQuiring Knowledge in Speech, Language and Hearing, 5*, 55–58.

Pound, C., Duchan, J., Penman, T., Hewitt, A., & Parr, S. (2007). Communication access to organisations: Inclusionary practices for people with aphasia. *Aphasiology, 21*, 23–38.

Prigatano, G., Roueche, J., & Fordyce, D. (1985). Nonaphasic language disturbances after closed head injury. *Language Sciences, 7*, 217–229.

Productivity Commission. (2005). *Economic implications of an ageing Australia*. Canberra: Australian Government Productivity Commission.

Pucci, E., Bellardinelli, N., Borsetti, G., & Giuliani, G. (2003). Relatives' attitudes towards informing patients about the diagnosis of Alzheimer's disease. *Journal of Medical Ethics, 29*, 51–54.

Ramig, L., Sapir, S., Countryman, S., Salwas, A., O'Brien, C., Hoehn, M., et al. (2001). Intensive voice treatment (LSVT®) for patients with Parkinson's disease: A 2 year follow up. *Journal of Neurology, Neurosurgery & Psychiatry, 71*, 493–498.

Rawls, J. (1971). *Theory of justice*. Oxford: Oxford University Press.

Reid-Proctor, G., Galin, K., & Cummings, M. (2001). Evaluation of legal competence in patients with frontal lobe injury. *Brain Injury, 15*, 377–386.

Ries, P. (1994). Prevalence and characteristics of persons with hearing trouble: United States, 1990–91. *Vital and Health Statistics, Series 10, No. 188*.

Robey, R. (1994). The efficacy of treatment for aphasic persons: A meta-analysis. *Brain and Language, 47*, 582–608.

Roseberry-McKibbin, C. (1997). Understanding Filipino families: A foundation for effective service delivery. *Journal of Speech-Language Pathology, 6*, 5–14.

Roseberry-McKibbin, C. (2000). 'Mirror, mirror on the wall': Reflections of a 'third-culture' American. *Communication Disorders Quarterly, 22*, 56–60.

Roseberry-McKibbin, C. (2004). *Multicultural students with special language needs* (2nd ed.). Oceanside, CA: Academic Communication.

Rosenthal, S. (1991). Communication skills in emotionally disturbed and nondisturbed adolescents. *Behavioral Disorders, 16*, 192–199.

Roulstone, S. (Ed.). (2007). *Prioritizing child health: Practice and principles*. London: Routledge.

Rowson, R. (2006). *Working ethics: How to be fair in a culturally complex world*. London: Jessica Kingsley.

Royal College of Speech and Language Therapists. (2005). *Speech and language therapy provision for people with dementia*. London: RCSLT.

Royal College of Speech and Language Therapists. (2006). *Communicating quality 3*. London: RCSLT.

Ruben, R. (2000). Redefining the survival of the fittest: Communication disorders in the 21st century. *The Laryngoscope, 110*, 241–245.

Sapir, S., Ramig, L., & Fox, C. (2006). The Lee Silvermann Voice Treatment® for voice, speech and other orofacial disorders in patients with Parkinson's disease. *Future Neurology*, 1, 563–570.

Savulescu, J. (2006). Conscientious objection in medicine. *British Medical Journal*, 332, 294–297.

Savulescu, J., Foddy, B., & Rogers, J. (2006). What should we say? *Journal of Medical Ethics*, 32, 7–12.

Scapoli, L., Palmieri, A., Martinelli, M., Pezzetti, F., Carinci, P., Tognon, M., et al. (2003). Strong evidence of linkage disequilibrium between polymorphisms at the IRF6 locus and nonsyndromic cleft lip with or without cleft palate in an Italian population. *The American Journal of Human Genetics*, 76, 180–183.

Schneider, G., & Snell, L. (2000). CARE: An approach for teaching ethics in medicine. *Social Science and Medicine*, 51, 1563–1567.

Schuklenk, U. (2006). Medical professionalism and ideological symbols in doctors' rooms. *Journal of Medical Ethics*, 32, 1–2.

Scottish Executive. (2000). *The same as you? A review of services for people with learning disabilities*. Edinburgh: The Scottish Government.

Seedhouse, D. (1998). *Ethics: The heart of healthcare* (2nd ed.). Chichester: Wiley.

Seedhouse, D. (2001). *Health: The foundations for achievement*. Chichester: Wiley.

Seedhouse, D. (2002a). Commitment to health: A shared ethical bond between professions. *Journal of Interprofessional Care*, 16, 249–260.

Seedhouse, D. (2002b). *Total health promotion: Mental health, rational fields and the quest for autonomy*. Chichester: Wiley.

Sharp, H., & Bryant, K. (2003). Ethical issues in dysphagia: When patients refuse assessment or treatment. *Seminars in Speech and Language*, 24, 285–299.

Sharp, H., & Genesen, L. (1996). Ethical decision-making in dysphagia management. *American Journal of Speech-Language Pathology*, 5, 15–22.

Shickle, D., & Chadwick, R. (1994). The ethics of screening: Is 'screeningitis' an incurable disease? *Journal of Medical Ethics*, 20, 12–18.

Sim, J. (1997). *Ethical decision making in therapy practice*. Oxford: Butterworth Heinemann.

Simmons-Mackie, N., & Damico, J. (1999). Social role negotiation in aphasia therapy: Competence, incompetence, and conflict. In D. Kovarsky, J. Duchan & M. Maxwell (Eds.), *Constructing (in)competence: Disabling valuations in clinical and social interaction* (pp. 313–341). Mahwah, NJ: Erlbaum.

Slote, M. (2007). *The ethics of care and empathy*. London: Routledge.

Snow, P. (in press). Child maltreatment, mental health and oral language competence: Inviting speech language pathology to the prevention table. *International Journal of Speech-Language Pathology*.

Sokol, D. (2006). Time to get streetwise: Why medical ethics needs doctors. *British Medical Journal*, 333, 1226.

Sokol, D. (2008). The 'four quadrants' approach to clinical ethics case analysis: An application and review. *Journal of Medical Ethics*, 34, 513–516.

Sokol, D., & Car, J. (2006). Patient confidentiality and telephone consultations: Time for a password. *Journal of Medical Ethics*, 32, 688–689.

South African Speech-Language-Hearing Association. (1997). *Code of ethics*. Auckland Park: South African Speech-Language-Hearing Association.

Speech Pathology Australia. (2000). *Code of ethics*. Melbourne: The Speech Pathology Association of Australia.

Speech Pathology Australia. (2001). *Competency-based occupational standards (CBOS) for speech pathologists: Entry level*. Melbourne: The Speech Pathology Association of Australia.

Speech Pathology Australia. (2002). *Speech Pathology Australia ethics education package*. Melbourne: The Speech Pathology Association of Australia.

Stauch, M. (2002). Comment on Re B (Adult: Refusal of medical treatment) [2002] 2 All England Reports 449. *British Medical Journal, 28*, 232–233.

Stranjalis, G. (1996). Ruptured cerebral aneurysm: Influence of specialist and trainee-performed operations on outcome. *Acta Neurochirurgica, 138*, 1067–1069.

Swanwick, R., & Tsverik, I. (2007). The role of sign language for deaf children with cochlear implants: Good practice in sign bilingual settings. *Deafness and Education International, 9*, 214–231.

Tate, G., & Turner, G. (1997). The code and the culture: Sign language interpreting – in search of the new breed's ethics. In F. Pöchhacker & M. Shlesinger (Eds.), *The interpreting studies reader* (2nd ed., pp. 372–383). New York: Routledge.

Theodoros, D. (2008). Telerehabilitation for service delivery in speech-language pathology. *Journal of Telemedicine and Telecare, 14*, 221–224.

Thompson, I., Melia, K., & Boyd, K. (2000). *Nursing ethics*. Edinburgh: Churchill Livingstone.

Togher, L. (2001). Discourse sampling in the 21st century. *Journal of Communication Disorders, 34*, 131–150.

Togher, L., Hand, L., & Code, C. (1997). Analysing discourse in the traumatic brain injury population: Telephone interactions with different communication partners. *Brain Injury, 11*, 169–189.

Togher, L., McDonald, S., Code, C., & Grant, S. (2004). Training communication partners of people with traumatic brain injury: A randomised controlled trial. *Aphasiology, 18*, 313–335.

Togher, L., Taylor, C., Smith, V., & Grant, S. (2006). Cognitive-communication skills of individuals following traumatic brain injury: A comparison across discourse genres. *Brain Impairment, 7*, 190–201.

Tronto, J. (1993). *Moral boundaries: A political argument for an ethic of care*. London: Routledge.

Turkstra, L., Coelho, C., & Ylvisaker, M. (2005). The use of standardized tests for individuals with cognitive-communication disorders. *Seminars in Speech and Language, 26*, 215–222.

Tweeddale, M. (2002). Grasping the nettle – what to do when patients withdraw their consent for treatment: (a clinical perspective on the case of Ms B). *Journal of Medical Ethics, 28*, 236–237.

United Nations. (1989). *Convention on the rights of the child*. Geneva: Office of the United Nations Commissioner for Human Rights.

United Nations. (1994a). *The Salamanca statement on principles, policy and practice in special needs education*. Paris: United Nations Educational Scientific and Cultural Organization.

United Nations. (1994b). *Standard rules on the equalization of opportunities for persons with disabilities*. Geneva: Office of the United Nations Commissioner for Human Rights.

United Nations. (2006). *Convention on the rights of persons with disabilities*. Geneva: Office of the United Nations Commissioner for Human Rights.

United Nations. (2007). *World population prospects: The 2006 revision*. New York: United Nations Department of Economic and Social Affairs.

van der Smagt-Duijnstee, M., Hamers, J., Abu-Saad, H., & Zuidhof, A. (2001). Relatives of hospitalized stroke patients: Their needs for information, counselling and accessibility. *Journal of Advanced Nursing, 33*, 307–315.

Viens, A., & Savulescu, J. (2004). Introduction to the Olivieri symposium. *Journal of Medical Ethics, 30*, 1–7.

Wiles, R., Pain, H., Buckland, S., & McLellan, L. (1998). Providing appropriate information to patients and carers following a stroke. *Journal of Advanced Nursing, 28*, 794–801.

Willer, B., & Corrigan, J. (1994). Whatever It Takes: A model for community-based services. *Brain Injury, 8*, 647–659.

Wilmot, S. (1997). *The ethics of community care*. London: Cassell.

Wilson, J., & Jungner, G. (1968). *Principles and practice of screening for disease*. Geneva: World Health Organization.

Wing, L., & Gould, J. (1979). Severe impairments of social interaction and associated abnormalities in children: Epidemiology and classification. *Journal of Autism and Developmental Disorders, 9*, 11–29.

World Health Organization. (2007). *International classification of functioning, disability and health. Version for children and youth: ICF-CY*. Geneva: World Health Organization.

Wright-St Clair, V., & Seedhouse, D. (2005). The moral context of practice and professional relationships. In G. Whiteford & V. Wright-St Clair (Eds.), *Occupation and practice in context* (pp. 16–33). Sydney: Elsevier Churchill Livingstone.

Yang-Lewis, T., & Moody, H. (1995). The forgetful mourner. *Hastings Centre Report, 25*, 32–33.

Ylvisaker, M., & Feeney, T. (1998). *Collaborative brain injury rehabilitation: Positive everyday routines*. San Diego: Singular.

Ylvisaker, M., Jacobs, H., & Feeney, T. (2003). Positive supports for people who experience behavioral and cognitive disability after brain injury: A review. *Journal of Head Trauma Rehabilitation, 18*, 7–32.

Index